Derouicha MATMOUR
Zakaria MERAD
Dalila MIRAOUI

Digestive system drugs

Derouicha MATMOUR
Zakaria MERAD
Dalila MIRAOUI

Digestive system drugs

Abstract of Therapeutic Chemistry

ScienciaScripts

Cover image: www.ingimage.com

This book is a translation from the original published under ISBN 978-620-6-71352-4.

Publisher:
Sciencia Scripts
is a trademark of
Dodo Books Indian Ocean Ltd. and OmniScriptum S.R.L publishing group

120 High Road, East Finchley, London, N2 9ED, United Kingdom
Str. Armeneasca 28/1, office 1, Chisinau MD-2012, Republic of Moldova, Europe
Managing Directors: Ieva Konstantinova, Victoria Ursu
info@omniscriptum.com

Printed at: see last page
ISBN: 978-620-8-57768-1

Contents

Foreword

The aim of *Therapeutic Chemistry* is to discover, develop and interpret the mechanism of action and the relationship between chemical structure and therapeutic activity of biologically active molecules obtained by chemical synthesis or hemi-synthesis. On an industrial scale, *Therapeutic Chemistry* deals with the manufacture and quality control of raw materials for pharmaceutical use, including active ingredients and excipients.

This *Compendium of Therapeutic Chemistry* comprises several volumes dealing with the different therapeutic classes of drugs, the sixth of which is devoted to *Drugs for the Digestive System.*

In each volume, *the Abrégé de Chimie Thérapeutique* describes the physio-pathology of the disease, the main drugs used, the main routes of chemical synthesis, the essential elements of quality control, the mechanism of action, the structure-activity relationship, the main indications and contraindications, and finally the undesirable effects.

The Compendium of Therapeutic Chemistry is intended for students of Pharmacy, Medicine and Pharmaceutical Chemistry, as well as post-graduate residents in Therapeutic Chemistry and Pharmacology, and drug professionals interested in the design, quality control and rational use of active ingredients.

Dr. Derouicha MATMOUR

Introduction to Volume 6

The sixth volume *of the Abrégé de Chimie Thérapeutique* is devoted to *Digestive System Drugs*, which are of particular clinical importance in the short- or long-term treatment of gastrointestinal pathologies that represent a major public health problem.
Four chapters are described in this volume, namely Antiemetic Drugs, Antispasmodic Drugs, Gastric Acidity Drugs and Laxative Drugs.
Each chapter deals successively with :
— General information on the therapeutic class and a physio-pathological overview of the disease concerned;
— History of discovery, pharmacochemical classification and main molecules marketed;
— Study of the leader for each class, i.e. its chemical synthesis and quality control according to the European Pharmacopoeia 9th edition;
— Molecular mechanism of action and study of the chemical structure-therapeutic activity relationship ;
- Main indications, contraindications, side effects, conclusions and outlook.
An alphabetical index is included at the end of the book, making it easier to search and access information by INN or proprietary name.

Dr. Derouicha MATMOUR

List of Authors

The following people took part in the preparation and writing of this book entitled: **"Volume 6: Medicinal products for the Digestive**

Dr. Derouicha MATMOUR
Dr. Zakaria MERAD
Dr. Dalila MIRAOUI
Sidi- Bel-Abbès Faculty of Medicine
Sidi- Faculty of Medicine
Bel-Abbès
Sidi- Faculty of Medicine
Bel-Abbès

Chapter 1

Anti-emetics

1. Introduction

Antiemetics are medicines that relieve nausea and vomiting.
The sensation of nausea is the result of a complex process in the body, which is why various medications have been developed to relieve nausea in different situations.

2. Pathophysiological background

2.1. Definition

Nausea and vomiting are essential protective defence processes by which humans and animals capable of vomiting tend to avoid ingesting and/or digesting potentially toxic substances.
Nausea is an unpleasant sensation experienced when you feel like vomiting, while vomiting is a physical event that consists of the forced expulsion of intestinal and gastric contents through the mouth.
Vomiting is often preceded by regurgitation, with the contents of the gastrointestinal tract being pushed back into the resophagus without the vomit being expelled.
Nausea and vomiting often occur in sequence, but this is not always the case. Sometimes severe nausea may be present without vomiting and, more rarely, vomiting may be present without nausea.
Nausea and vomiting can be triggered by several mechanisms (Figure 1).

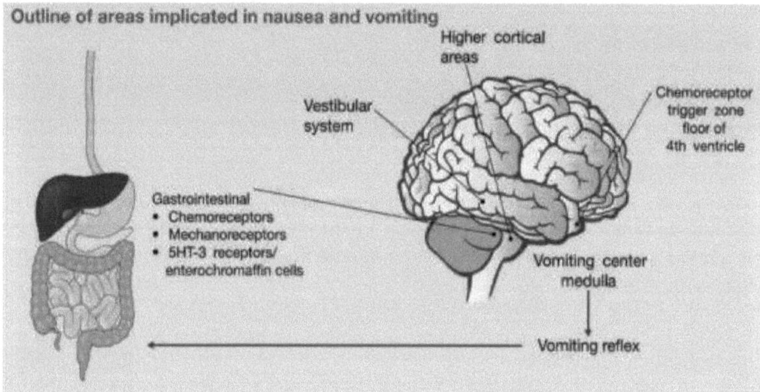

Figure 1: The different mechanisms involved in vomiting (Louise Denholm et al, 2021).

2.2. Central and peripheral sites of nausea and vomiting

Two key sites in the central nervous system are involved in the organisation of the vomiting reflex: the vomiting centre and the CTZ chemoreceptor trigger zone (Figure 2).

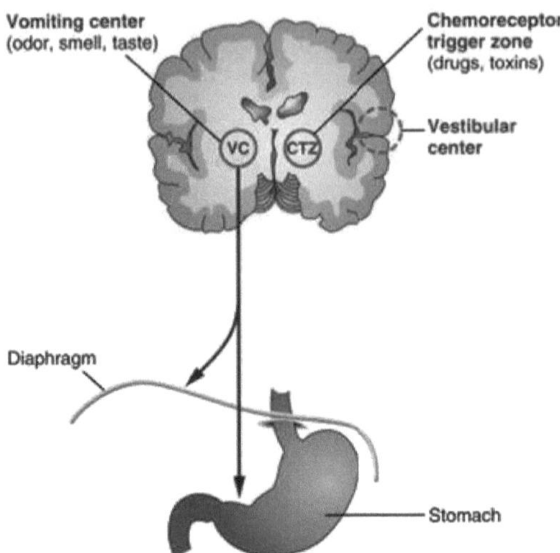

Figure 2. Key central sites involved in the regulation of emesis (McCuistion et al,2022).

Five key neurotransmitters are involved in the afferent response to these areas. These are histamine (H1 receptors), dopamine (D2), serotonin (5-HT3), acetylcholine (muscarinic) and neurokinin (substance P).

There are five key factors that trigger vomiting:

1. The presence of toxic substances in the lumen of the gastrointestinal tract
2. Visceral pathology
3. Vestibular disturbance
4. Stimulation of the central nervous system
5. Toxins in blood or cerebrospinal fluid

2.3. Vomiting centre

The vomiting centre is located in **the medulla oblongata**. It is unlikely to represent a distinct area of the brain and is thought to encompass the nucleus of the tractus solitarius. It receives afferent signals from the superior zones, the **vagus nerve, the vestibular nuclei** and **the CTZ** (Figure 3).

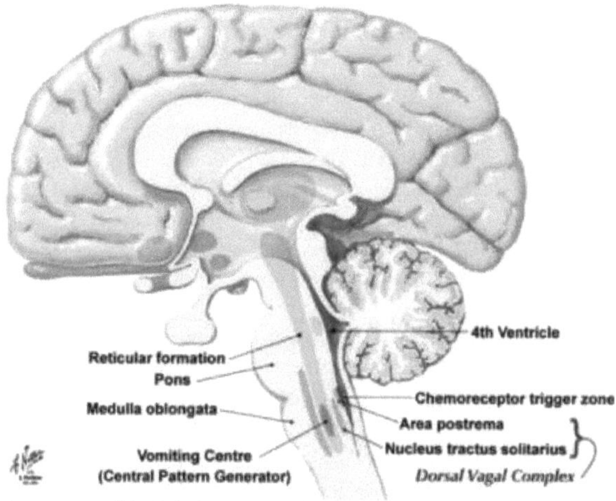

Figure 3: Vomiting centre (McCuistion et al, 2022).

2.4. Chemoreceptor trigger zone

The **CTZ**, or "**area postrema**", lies at the bottom of **the fourth ventricle**. Interestingly, this area lies **outside the cerebrospinal fluid** (CSF), although it is particularly good at **detecting hormones** and **toxins** in the **CSF** and **bloodstream** thanks to its dense **capillary network** and fenestrated epithelium.

Drug-induced vomiting is common. CTZ may be stimulated by the drugs themselves or by metabolites produced when the drug is broken down.

Medicines can also affect intestinal motility, leading to stimulation of muscle receptors, and can irritate the gastric mucosa, causing nausea and vomiting.

The drugs most commonly involved **are opiates, volatile anaesthetics** and **cytotoxics**.

2.5. Vagal afferent pathways

The vagal afferent pathways **are major peripheral emetic nerves** that play an important role in emesis **in response to emetic stimuli** in **the gastrointestinal tract**.

In response to peripheral emetic stimuli, gastrointestinal vagal afferent fibres transmit information about the physiological state of the gastrointestinal tract to the dorsal vagal complex, and activation of vagal afferents is involved in the generation of vomiting.

2.6. Gastrointestinal tract

In the gastrointestinal tract, **enterochromaffin cells** synthesise over **90%** of the body's 5-hydroxytryptamine (serotonin, 5- HT), as well as large quantities of **substance P** (SP), **both** of which **are essential** for **gastrointestinal motility**, **nausea** and **vomiting**.

Emetogenic **chemical**, **mechanical** or **neurological** stimuli induce the release of 5-HT and/or SP by enterochromaffin cells in a **calcium** (Ca^{2+})**-dependent** manner.

Following their release, 5-HT, and probably SP, stimulate **their** corresponding **emetic receptors** (serotonin 5-HT3 receptors and neurokinin substance P NK1 receptors, respectively), which are present on **the vagal afferents** that cause nausea and vomiting.

As 5-HT in the bloodstream is ionised at physiological pH, it is unlikely to reach the emetic nuclei of the brainstem; however, an active substance P transport mechanism is present in the brainstem.

2.7. Receptors involved in emesis induction

Exogenous stimuli, particularly emetogenic cancer chemotherapy, bacterial toxins in the intestine, viral and fungal infections, food poisoning, epigastric radiation, various drugs and movement, cause vomiting, which is often, but not always, accompanied by nausea.

They act either directly at their target site(s), or indirectly via the release of emetic neurotransmitters/mediators, to activate the corresponding emetic receptors, including serotonin type 3 (5-HT3), neurokinin 1 (NK1), dopamine D2 and D3, mu and kappa opioYdes, muscarin M1, and histamine H1, many of which are located both in the periphery (e.g. gastrointestinal tract, vagal afferents) and in the dorsal vagal complex of the brainstem (area postrema)

With the exception of some ion channel-coupled receptors, such as 5-HT3 and transient receptor for vanilloid potential type 1 (TRPV1), many emetic receptors belong to the G protein-coupled receptor (GPCR) family (Figure 4).

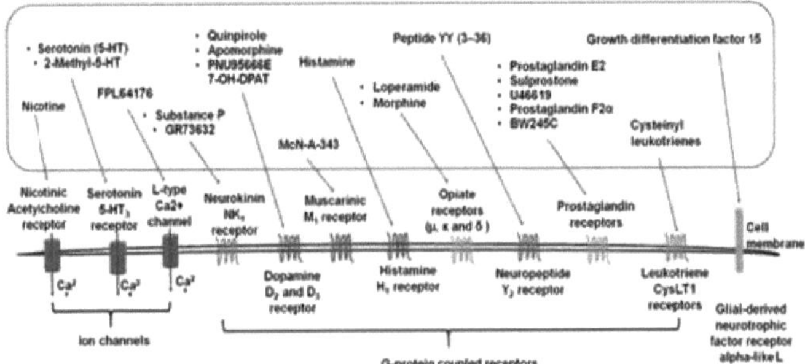

Figure 4. Different receptors involved in the regulation of emesis (Weixia Zhong et al, 2021).

2.7.1. Serotonin receptors

Serotonin receptors can be classified into seven major families (5-HT1-7), which are G protein-coupled transmembrane receptors, with the exception of the 5-HT3 receptor, which belongs to the ion channel family (Figure 5).

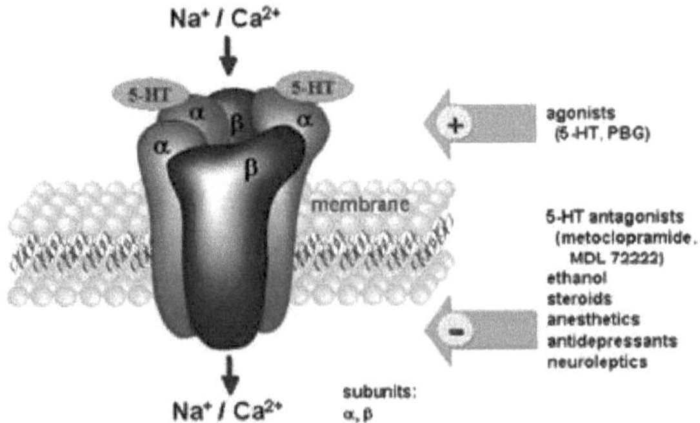

Figure 5: 5HT3 receptor (Jutta Walstab et al , 2010).

As an ion channel, activation of the 5-HT3 receptor induces rapid excitatory postsynaptic potentials and rapid depolarisation of serotonergic neurons, leading to an increase in intracellular $Ca^{(2+)}$) concentration, which causes the release of various neurotransmitters and/or emetic peptides (e.g. dopamine, cholecystokinin, glutamate, acetylcholine, substance P or 5-HT itself), as well as an increase in intracellular Ca^{2+} concentration⁾

2.7.2. Substance P NK1 neurokinin receptor (NK1R)

Substance P is one of the members of the structurally related mammalian tachykinin peptide family, comprising neurokinin A, neurokinin B and N-terminally extended forms of neurokinin A, such as neuropeptide K and neurokinin g.

Mammalian tachykinins activate three specific membrane-associated neurokinin receptors, known as NK1, NK2 and NK3, which belong to the G protein-coupled receptor superfamily.

Substance P appears to be the endogenous ligand for NK1 receptors and plays a major role in the induction of emesis, particularly during the delayed phase of emesis induced by cancer chemotherapy.

Both NK1R neurokinins and substance P are expressed in central and peripheral emetic sites, including the emetic nuclei of the dorsal vagal complex of the brainstem, as well as in vagal afferents, where central NK1Rs play a major role and peripheral NK1Rs a minor role in emesis induction.

2.7.3. D2/3 dopamine receptors

Dopamine is a monoaminergic neurotransmitter that produces its various physiological effects by activating two classes of G protein-coupled membrane receptors, namely D1like dopamine receptors (D1 and D5) and D2like dopamine receptors (D2, D3 and D4).

To date, numerous animal studies have implicated D2 and D3 dopamine receptors in mediating emesis, while selective D1/D4/D5 dopamine receptor agonists lack emetic properties.

Dopamine, its pro-emetic receptors (dopamine D2/3) and/or their mRNA are well distributed throughout the emetic reflex arc, including the dorsal vagal complex (area postrema, nucleus tractus solitarius, dorsal motor nucleus of the vagus nerve), vagal nerves, gastrointestinal tract and enteric nervous system.

In fact, dopaminergic tissue levels and turnover increase in the brainstem and jejunum of the mouse pup during the early and delayed phases of emesis following cisplatin administration in the mouse pup emesis model.

2.7.4. Acetylcholine receptors

Acetylcholine plays an important physiological role. It activates nicotinic receptor ion channels, as well as G protein-coupled muscarinic receptors, which are made up of five subtypes, M1-M5.

Clinically used drugs that inhibit the metabolism of acetylcholine, such as choline esterase inhibitors (e.g. donepezil, galantamine, rivastigmine, etc.), cause vomiting in humans.

Stimulation of muscarinic receptors also leads emesis; however, the precise role each of the five muscarinic subtypes in emesis has not yet been fully defined.

2.7.5. Histamine H1 receptor

Significant preclinical evidence indicates that vestibular hyperactivity triggers activation of the histaminergic neuronal system during motion sickness, ultimately stimulating histamine H1 receptors in the brainstem and inducing vomiting. In fact, intracerebroventricular injections of histamine cause vomiting, which is suppressed by bilateral removal of the area postrema or prior treatment antihistamines.

Histamine also has a peripheral emetic component, since its release from intestinal mast cells contributes to vomiting in mice in response to food poisoning caused by staphylococcal enterotoxins.

2.7.6. Other

- Opiate receptors
- Neuropeptide Y2 receptors
- Growth and differentiation factor 15 receptor (GDF15)
- eicosanoYde receptors

— Prostaglandins.

3. History of the discovery of antiemetics

The desire to identify antiemetic drugs most likely **originated in the desire to** combat **seasickness**, with references to treatments in **classical Greek** and **Roman literature** and, more recently, **Shakespeare**.

These and subsequent attempts to block nausea and vomiting before and during the Second World War (WWII, 1939-1945) were largely based on **traditional**, **historical** and unproven **remedies** for seasickness, with over 40 treatments identified on the basis of publications in the Lancet between 1828 and 1928.

The only substances recognised in antiquity and **before the Second World War** whose **effectiveness was** subsequently **demonstrated atropine** and **hyoscine.**

In **1976, a series of** largely fortuitous **developments** led to identification of **four classes** of antiemetic drugs (Gibbs 1976):

1. **Anticholinergic drugs** (which have subsequently been shown to act as antagonists of M3 and M5 muscarinic receptors);
2. **Antihistamines** (which were later shown to act mainly as antagonists of histamine H1 receptors, but also of muscarinic receptors);
3. **Phenothiazine derivatives** (which act as dopamine D2 receptor antagonists, but also on other receptors);
4. ***Metoclopramide***, a drug derived from the local anaesthetic procainamide (initially described as a D2 receptor antagonist before other activities were discovered a few years later.

DOMPERIDONE was identified in **1974** as a member of the **butyrophenone** class of compounds. The drug was described as similar to metoclopramide and marketed in **1982** for the prevention of nausea and vomiting, including those induced by cancer chemotherapy.

Subsequent studies have shown that DOMPERIDONE has a similar affinity for human D2 and D3 receptors.

Baker et al (1979) found that *DEXAMETHASONE* (10 mg) reduced emesis induced by various cytotoxic anticancer drugs, but it was suggested that the associated euphoria played a role. A pilot clinical study using *METHYLPREDNISOLONE* to inhibit prostaglandin release (Rich et al., 1980) also **showed efficacy** (in combination with chlorpromazine or prochlorperazine) in patients receiving **cisplatin-based** treatment.

Subsequent studies using high doses of dexamethasone in patients receiving cisplatin alone or in combination with other cytotoxic drugs reported impressive responses with excellent or good control of nausea and vomiting in 50% of patients who had failed standard antiemetics and 71% in patients who had not previously received antiemetics.

In the early **1970s**, isolated reports of reduced nausea and vomiting **in marijuana users** undergoing chemotherapy for Hodgkin's disease led to clinical evaluation of **the antiemetic use of marijuana** and THC (Δ-9-tetrahydrocannabinol, the main psychoactive constituent) in cancer patients undergoing chemotherapy.

They act as a receptor agonist, activating CB1 receptors in the dorsal vagal complex of the brainstem and the visceral cortex. The clinical potential of selective CB1 receptor agonists remains to be assessed.

Since the discovery of 5-HT3 and NK1 receptor antagonists, there has been a major advance in the treatment of nausea and vomiting.

4. Classification of antiemetics

The different classes of antiemetics **target different pro-emetic regulatory pathways** to relieve nausea and vomiting. Some target more than one of these pathways.

The **five main classes of antiemetics** are :
— Dopamine antagonists ;
— Serotonin antagonists ;
— Neurokinin antagonist ;
— Histamine antagonists ;
— Acetylcholine antagonists.

Cannabinoid agonists, corticosteroids and **benzodiazepines** also have antiemetic effects.

5. Dopamine antagonists

They raise **the threshold for the** vomiting **reflex** by **inhibiting type 2** (D2) **receptors centrally** in the chemoreceptor trigger zone and **peripherally** in the gastrointestinal tract. They are therefore useful in the prevention and treatment of vomiting associated with drugs and toxins in the bloodstream.

There are currently several **chemical classes of** D2 dopamine receptor antagonists, such as :

— **Phenothiazines** (e.g. chlorpromazine) ;
— **Butyrophenones** (e.g. haloperidol) ;
— **Benzamides** (for example, metoclopramide, which also blocks 5-HT3 receptors).

They are used clinically to prevent vomiting caused by a variety of emetic stimuli, including **radiotherapy**, **viral gastroenteritis**, **food-induced vomiting** and **post-operative vomiting**, as well **as prophylaxis** for **cancer patients** receiving chemotherapy with low emetogenic potential (**table I**).

Table I. Main dopamine antagonists.

Chemical class	Molecule DCI	Trade name and pharmaceutical form	Chemical structure and scientific name
Benzamides	Métoclopramide	***PRIMPERAN®*** Solution buvable Solution injectable á 10mg/ 2mL Comprimé sécable á 10 mg	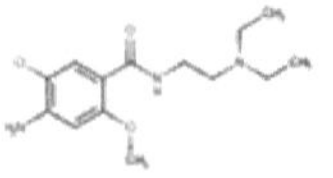 4-amino-5-chloro-N-[2-(diéthyl amino) éth yl]-2-méthoxy benz amide
	Alizapride	***PLITICAN®*** Comprimé á 50 mg	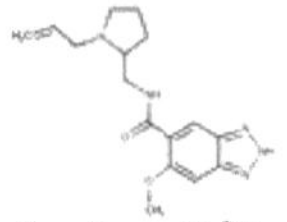 6-methoxy-N-{[1-(pro p-2-en-1-yl)pyrrolidin-2-yl]methyl}-2H-1,2,3-benzotriazole-5-carbo xamide
Benzimidazoles	Dompéridone	***MOTILIUM®*** Comprimé á 10 mg Solution buvable	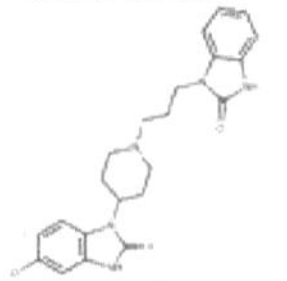 5-chloro-1-{1-[3-(2-oxo-2,3-dihydro-1H-1,3-benzodiazol-1-yl) propyl] piperidin-4-yl} -2,3-dihydro-1H-1,3-benzodiazol-2-one
Phénothiazines	Prochlorperazine	***COMPAZINE®*** Comprimé á 5mg	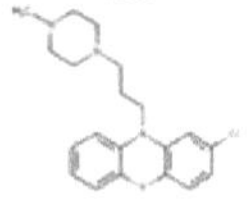 2-chloro-10-[3-(4-met hylpiperazin-1-yl)pro pyl]-10H-phenothiazin

Table I. Main dopamine antagonists (continued).

Chemical class	Molecule DCI	Trade name and pharmaceutical form	Chemical structure and scientific name
Phénothiazines	Prochlorperazine	**COMPAZINE®** Comprimé á 5mg	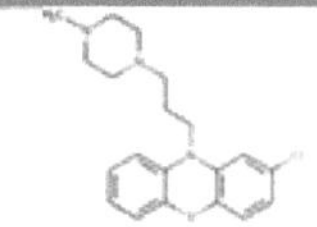 2-chloro-10-[3-(4-methylpiperazin-1-yl) propyl]-10H-phenothiazine
	METOPIMAZINE	***VOGALENE®*** *Solution buvable* *Solution injectable á 10mg/1mL* *Comprimé á* *7,5 mg et 10 mg*	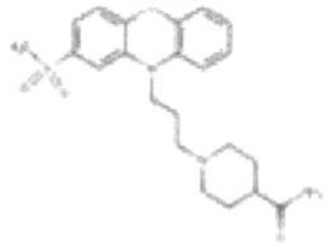 1-[3-(2-methanesulfonyl-10H-phenothiazin-10-yl)propyl]piperidine-4-carboxamide
Butyrophénones	Dropéridol	***DROLEPTAN®*** Solution injectable á 1,25 mg/2,5 ml	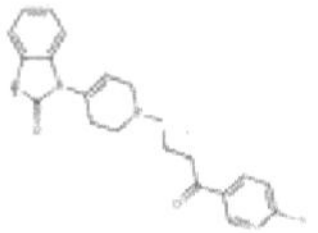 1-{1-[4-(4-fluoropheny l)-4-oxobutyl]-1,2,3,6-tetrahydro pyridin-4-yl}-2,3-dihydro-1H-1,3 -benzodiazol-2-one
	Halopéridol	***HALDOL®*** *Goutte buvable*	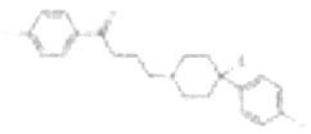 4-[4-(4-chlorophenyl)-4-hydroxy piperidin-1-yl]-1-(4-fluorophenyl) butan-1-one

Table I. Main dopamine antagonists (continued).

Chemical class	Molecule INN	Trade name and pharmaceutical form	Structure chemical and scientific name

Antipsychotiques atypiques	Olanzapine	**ZYPREXA®** Comprimé á 5mg et 10 mg	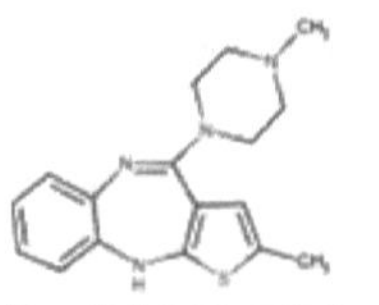 2-methyl-4-(4-methylpiperazin-1-yl)-10*H*-thieno[2,3b][1,5]benzodiazepine

5.1. Study of the lead partner

Metoclopramide: *PRIMPERAN®*

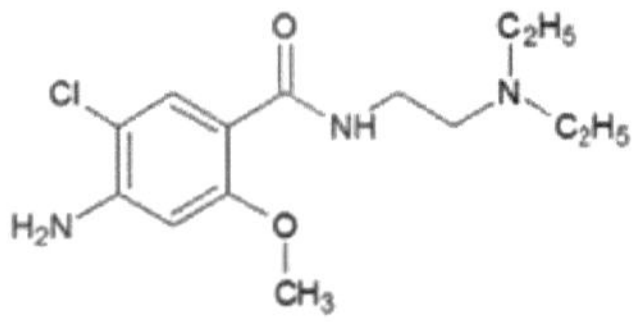

Figure 6. Structure of Metoclopramide.

5.1.1. Chemical synthesis

The action of nitric acid on 2-aminotoluene leads to the nitro derivative which, through the action of sodium nitrite in a hydrochloric medium, gives diazonium arene salt. The latter is transformed into the corresponding phenol in the presence of water (aromatic nucleophilic substitution).

The action of dimethyl sulphate in a basic medium gives an ether derivative, potassium permanganate provides the carboxylic acid which is converted to acid by thionyl chloride.

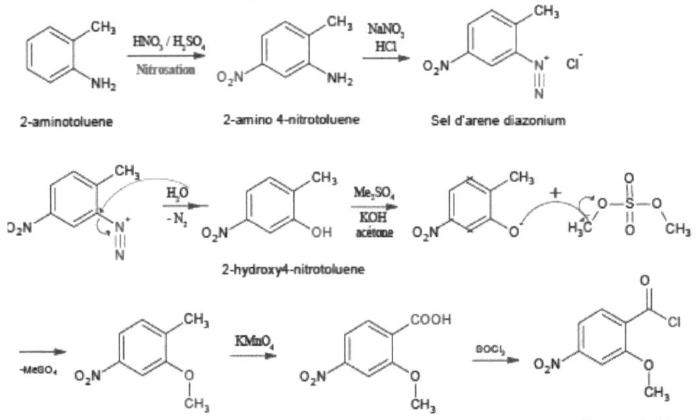

2-aminotoluene —(HNO_3 / H_2SO_4, Nitrosation)→ 2-amino 4-nitrotoluene —($NaNO_2$, HCl)→ Sel d'arene diazonium

—(H_2O, $-N_2$)→ 2-hydroxy4-nitrotoluene —(Me_2SO_4, KOH, acétone)→ —($-MeSO_4$)→ Ether —($KMnO_4$)→ Acide 2-methoxy 4-nitro benzoique —($SOCl_2$)→ Chlorure d'acide

Figure 7. Chemical synthesis of metoclopramide.

Amidation with *N*,N-diethylaminoethylamine gives intermediate I, which undergoes catalytic hydrogenation to an aromatic amine.

Metoclopramide is finally obtained by bubbling chlorine gas in acetic acid-acetic anhydride medium (SE Ar).

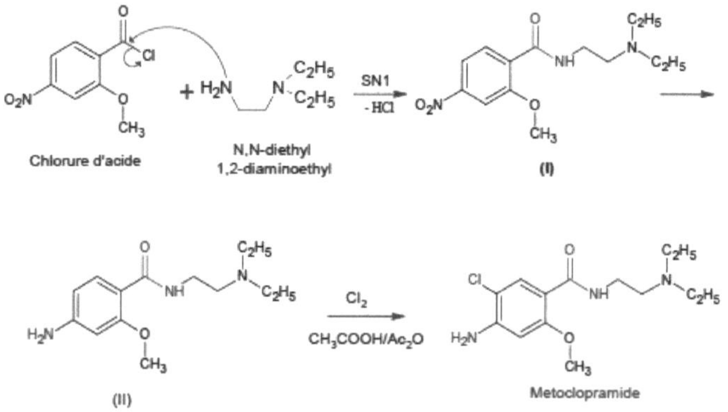

Figure 8. Chemical synthesis of Metoclopramide (continued).

5.1.2. Analytical control

1. Physico-chemical properties

Metoclopramide is a fine, white or approximately white powder. It is practically insoluble in water, fairly soluble or sparingly soluble in ethanol and sparingly soluble in methylene chloride. Metoclopramide is polymorphic.

2. Identification

- Melting point: 145°C to 149°C.
- Infrared absorption spectrophotometry

3. Test

- Related substances
- Appearance of the solution
- Loss on drying
- Sulphuric ash

4. Dosage

Titration by potentiometry.

5.1.3. Pharmacokinetics

Metoclopramide is rapidly and **well absorbed** from the gastrointestinal tract, and peak plasma concentrations are reached approximately **1** to **2 hours** after oral administration. Metoclopramide **is fat-soluble**, giving it a long half-life and volume of distribution. Its half-life can vary from **4.5 hours** to **8.8 hours.**

The volume of distribution is high (around 3.5 L/kg).

Metoclopramide is metabolised by **oxidation**, mainly via cytochrome **P450 2D6** (CYP2D6), by glucuronide and by conjugation with sulphate. Approximately 85% of the radioactivity of an oral dose is recovered **in the urine**.

6. Serotonin antagonists

There is significant clinical evidence that **first-generation** (e.g. ondansetron, granisetron, dolasetron) and **second-generation** (e.g. palonosetron) 5-HT3 antagonists attenuate **the first phase of emesis** induced **by cancer chemotherapy**, where **serotonin** plays **a major emetic role**.

Because of their serotonergic action, these drugs can cause **serotonin syndrome**, especially if used at the same time as other serotonergic drugs (table II).

Table II. Main serotonin antagonists.

Molecule INN	Trade name and pharmaceutical form	Chemical structure and scientific name
Ondansétron	***ZOPHREN®*** Solution injectable à 2 mg /mL Comprimé à 4mg et 8 mg	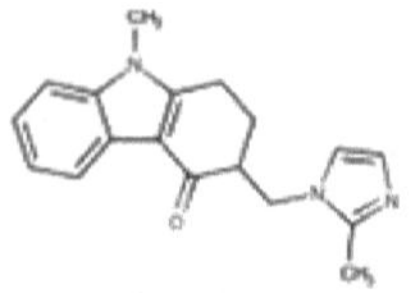 9-methyl-3-[(2-methyl-1H-imidazol-1-yl)methyl]-2,3,4,9-tetrahydro-1H-carbazol-4-one
Granisétron	***KYTRIL®*** Comprimé à 1mg et 2 mg Solution injectable à 3 mg /3mL	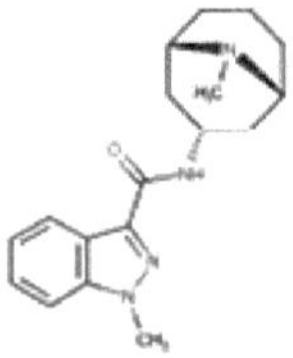 1-methyl-N-[(1R,3r,5S)-9-methyl-9-azabicyclo [3.3.1]nonan-3-yl]-1H-indazole-3-carboxamide
Tropisetron	***TROPISETRON®*** Solution injectable à 5 mg /5mL	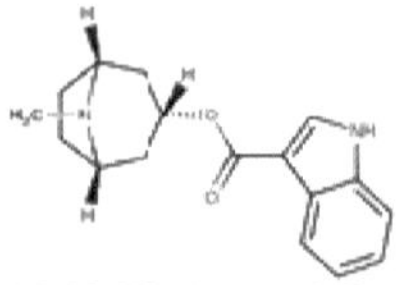 (1R,3S,5S)-8-methyl-8-aza bicyclo[3.2.1]octan-3-yl 1H-indole-3-carboxy late
Palonosétron	**PALONOSETRON ACCORD®** Solution injectable à 0,25 mg /5 mL	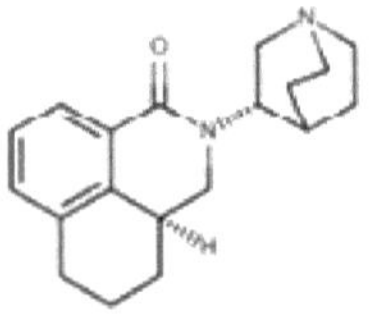 (5S)-3-[(3S)-1-azabicyclo[2.2.2]octan-3-yl]-3-azatricyclo[7.3.1.$0^{5,13}$]trideca-1(12),9(13),10-trien-2-one

6.1. Study of the lead partner

Ondansetron: *ZOPHREN®* (in French)

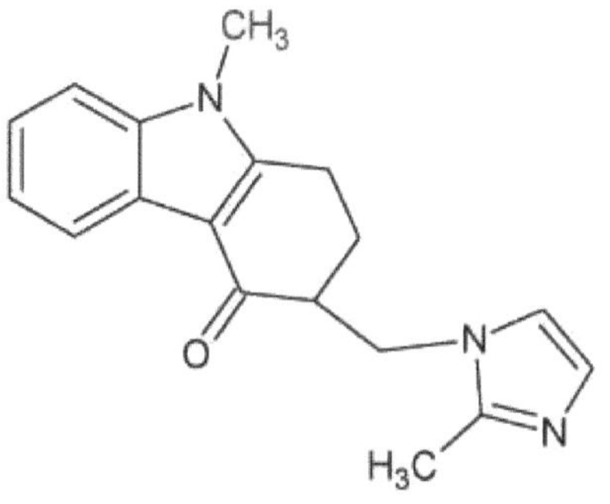

Figure 9. Structure de l'Ondansétron.

Ondansetron, considered to be the reference antiemetic, is an example of a highly selective 5-HT3 receptor antagonist that acts on the central and peripheral nervous systems. It has no cardiovascular or respiratory effects and is not sedating.

6.1.1. Chemical synthesis

Condensation of 2-bromoaniline with cyclohexane-1,3-dione gives the bromo enaminone, which is N-methylated with iodomethane and NaH to give the tertiary enaminone. Treatment of the latter with the triphenylphosphine-palladium acetate/NHCO3 complex or palladium acetate in acetonitrile **gives the carbazolone**.

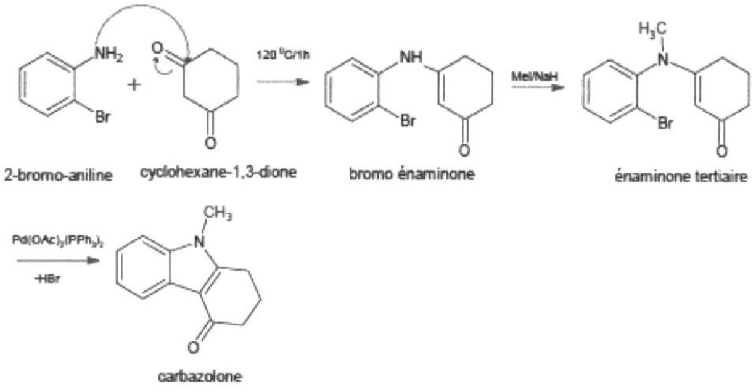

Figure 10. Synthesis of Ondansetron.

Treatment of carbazolone with sodium metal in EtOH/dioxane and diethyl oxalate yields an ethoxallyl derivative, which is then converted to a glyoxylic acid lactone.

Coupling glyoxylic acid lactone with 2-methylimidazol using **benzyltriethylammonium** chloride in CHCl3/H2O gives glyoxylate, which is converted to the target product by further reaction with 2-methylimidazol in dioxane and final treatment with HCl.

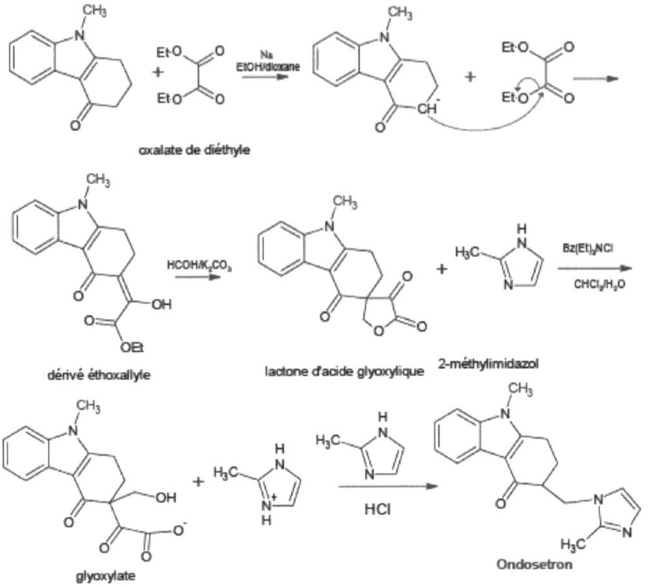

Figure 11. Synthesis of Ondansetron (continued).

6.1.2. Analytical control

1. Physico-chemical properties

Ondansetron is a white or approximately white powder. It is soluble in water, soluble in methanol, fairly soluble in 96% ethanol and sparingly soluble in methylene chloride.

2. Identification

- Infrared absorption spectrophotometry

3. Test

- Related substances
- Sulphuric ash

4. Dosage

Liquid chromatography

6.1.3. Pharmacokinetics

Ondansetron is absorbed from the gastrointestinal tract and undergoes limited first-pass metabolism.

The volume of distribution of ondansetron is approximately 160 litres.

Ondansetron is a substrate for human hepatic cytochrome P450 enzymes, notably CYP1A2, CYP2D6 and CYP3A4.

Ondansetron is extensively metabolised and excreted in the urine and faeces.

7. Neurokinin antagonist

Clinically, NK1R antagonists (such as aprepitant, netupitant and rolapitant) are recommended for the suppression of second-phase vomiting induced by highly emetogenic cancer chemotherapy.

In fact, they are one of the main components of the "prophylactic antiemetic triple therapy", along with one of the 5-HT3 receptor antagonists described above and dexamethasone.

Baseline studies have indicated that NK1R antagonists behave as broad-spectrum antiemetics and are also clinically effective against postoperative nausea and vomiting; however, they are not recommended in patients on contraceptives, as aprepitant reduces the efficacy of oral contraceptives (Table III).

Tableau III. Main NK1R antagonists.

Molecule INN	Trade name and pharmaceutical form	Chemical structure and scientific name
Aprepitant	***EMEND®*** Gélule à 80 mg et 125 mg	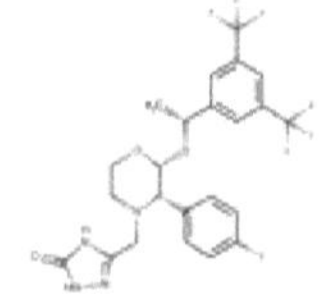 3-{[(2R,3S)-2-[(1R)-1-[3,5-bis(trifluoro methyl)phenyl] ethoxy]-3-(4-fluorophenyl) morpholin-4-yl]methyl}-4,5 -dihydro-1H-1,2,4-triazol-5-one
Fosaprepitant la prodrogue de l'aprépitant	***EMEND®*** *Solution injectable* à 150 mg	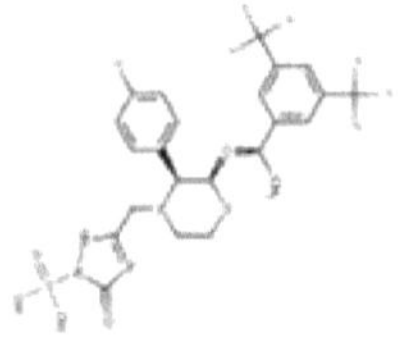 (3-{[(2R,3S)-2-[(1R)-1-[3,5-bis(trifluoro methyl)phenyl] ethoxy]-3-(4-fluorophenyl) morpholin-4-yl]methyl}-5-oxo-2,5-dihydro-1H-1,2,4-triazol-1-yl)phosphonic acid
Netupitant	***AKYNZEO®*** *Solution injectable à 300 mg / 0,5 mg* (Netupitant/Palonosétron)	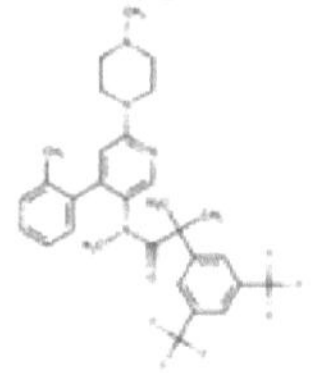 2-[3,5-bis(trifluoromethyl) phenyl]-N,2-dimethyl-N-[4-(2-me thylphenyl)-6-(4-me thyl pipera zin-1-yl)pyridin -3-yl]propan amide

3.1. Study of the lead partner

Aprepitant: *EMEND®*

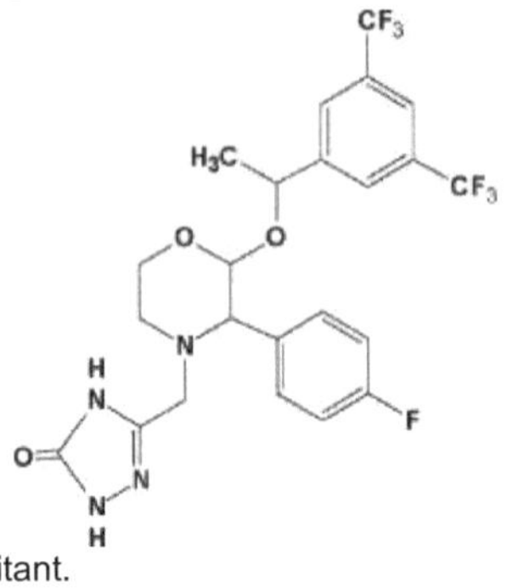

Figure 11. Structure of Aprepitant.

3.1.1. Chemical synthesis

N-benzylhydroxyethylamine reacted with **ethyl oxalate** to give morpholinedione. Selective reduction of the latter by **lithium tri-secbutylborohydride** leads to an intermediate (I), which by the action of **trifluoroacetic anhydride** (ATFA) gives access to trifluoroacetate, which is treated without isolation by **3,5-bis-(trifluoromethyl)phen-1-ylethanol** to give intermediate (II).

The action of 4-fluorophenylmagnesium bromide provides the imine by a complex mechanism (first addition of the organomagnesium to the carbonyl to give a tertiary alcohol, followed by hydrogen debenzylation in the presence of carbon palladium and para-toluenesulphonic acid and finally dehydration favoured by steric hindrance).

Reduction followed by salification (HCl) leads to the secondary amine. The action of N-methoxycarbonyl-2-chloroacetamidrazone leads to a cyclised compound transformed into aprepitant by heat treatment.

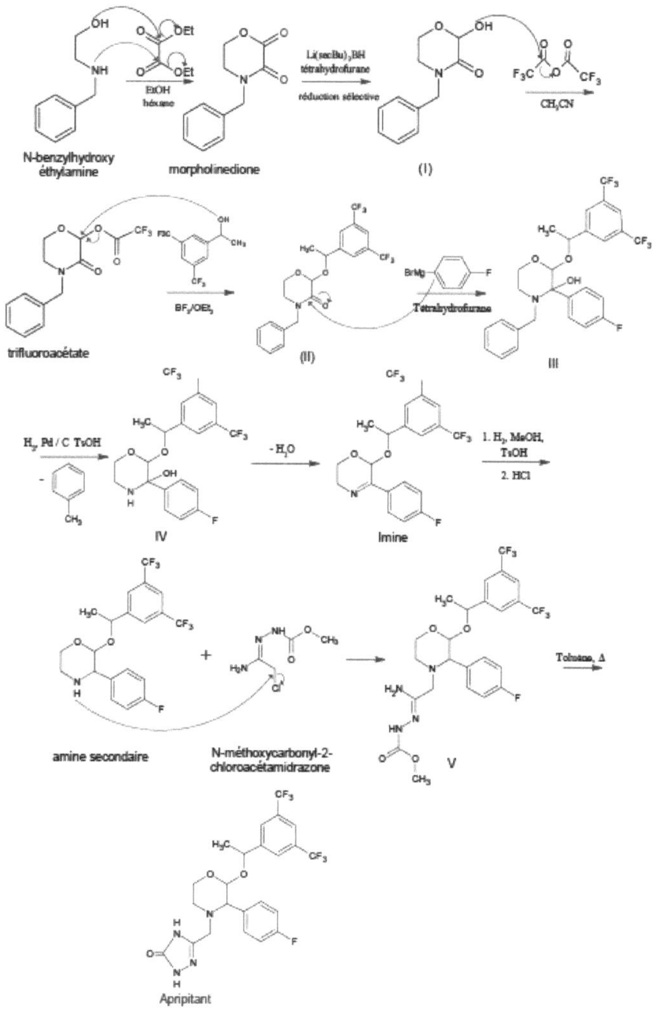

Figure 12. Chemical synthesis of Aprepitant.

3.1.2. Analytical control

1. Physico-chemical properties

Aprepitant is a white or almost white powder. It is very slightly soluble in water, fairly soluble in anhydrous ethanol and practically insoluble in heptane. Aprepitant is polymorphic.

2. Identification

- Infrared absorption spectrophotometry
- Specific rotation: + 66.0 to + 70.0

3. Test

- Related substances
- Sulphuric ash
- Water

4. Dosage

Liquid chromatography.

3.1.3. Pharmacokinetics

The mean absolute oral bioavailability of aprepitant is approximately 60-65%, with a volume of distribution of 70 L.

Protein binding is reported as >95%.

Aprepitant is mainly metabolised by CYP3A4, with minor metabolism by CYP1A2 and CYP2C19.

Aprepitant is eliminated mainly by metabolism; it is not excreted by the kidneys, with a half-life of 9-13 hours.

3.1.4. Histamine antagonists

Histamine H1-receptor blockers, such as dimenhydrinate and diphenhydramine, are antiemetic agents commonly used to combat the nausea and vomiting associated with motion sickness.

It is important to note that many H1-receptor blockers have anticholinergic properties that block muscarinic receptors, which may also contribute to their antiemetic effects (Table IV).

Table IV. Main H1 receptor antagonists.

Molecule INN	Trade name and pharmaceutical form	Chemical structure and scientific name
Cyclizine	**CYCLIZINE®** Comprimé à 50 mg	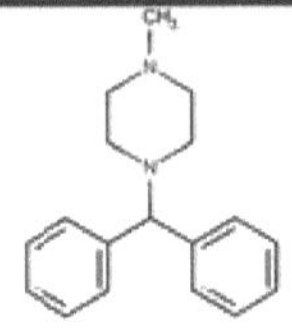 1-(diphenylmethyl)-4-methylpiperazine
Prométhazine	***PHENERGAN®*** *Solution buvable*	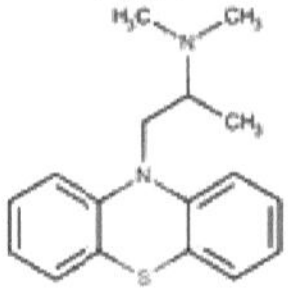 dimethyl[1-(10H-phenothiazin-10-yl)propan-2-yl]amine

Table IV. Main H1 receptor antagonists (continued).

Molecule INN	Trade name and pharmaceutical form	Chemical structure and scientific name
Pheniramine	***PHENIRAMINE MALEATE®*** Solution injectable	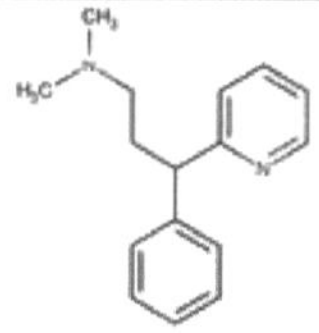 dimethyl[3-phenyl-3-(pyridin-2-yl)propyl]amine
Doxylamine	**CARIBAN®** Comprimé à 15 mg et 25 mg	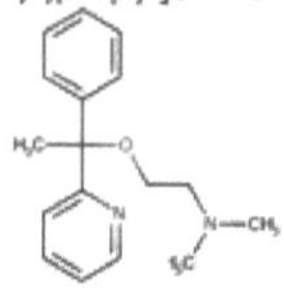 dimethyl({2-[1-phenyl-1-(pyridin-2-yl)ethoxy]ethyl})amine

9. Acetylcholine antagonists

Currently available non-selective muscarinic receptor antagonists, such as scopolamine and atropine, which also block M1 receptors, are used for the prevention of nausea and vomiting caused by motion sickness. Transdermal scopolamine is also effective against postoperative nausea and vomiting (table V).

Table V. Main acetylcholine antagonists.

Molecule INN	Trade name and pharmaceutical form	Chemical structure and scientific name
Scopolamine	**SCOPODERM®** Dispositif transdermique á 1 mg/72 h	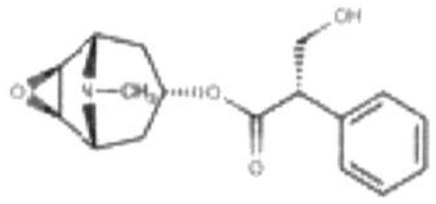 (1R,2R,4S,5S,7S)-9-methyl-3-oxa-9-azatricyclo[3.3.1.0^{ 2,4 }]nonan-7-yl (2S)-3-hydrox y-2-phenylpropanoate

10. Other

10.1. Steroids

Steroids such as ***DEXAMETHASONE*** are also useful as antiemetics, and antiemetic effects occur with all glucocorticoids. However, the mechanism by which they achieve this is not clear.

Combination with 5-HT3 antagonists results in a reduction in serotonin concentrations in the intestine, with increased sensitivity of 5-HT3 receptors to antiemetics.

10.2. Benzodiazepines

Lorazepam: acts on the chemoreceptor trigger zone, suppressing dopamine activity.

10.3. CannabinoYdes

Such as Tetrahydrocannabinol, they activate CB1 cannabinoid receptors (inhibitors) in the central and peripheral nervous systems to modulate the release of neurotransmitters. However, they are not used.

11. Conclusion and outlook

Antiemetic drugs are a crucial class of medicines used to treat and prevent nausea and vomiting. They work by targeting various receptors in the brain and gastrointestinal tract that are responsible for inducing vomiting. These drugs are commonly used in patients undergoing chemotherapy, radiotherapy or surgery, as well as those suffering from motion sickness or other conditions that cause nausea and vomiting.

There are different types of antiemetic drugs, including serotonin antagonists, dopamine antagonists, neurokinin-1 receptor antagonists and antihistamines. Each type of medication has a unique mechanism of action and is used for different types of nausea and vomiting.

Although antiemetic drugs are generally safe and effective, they can cause side effects such as drowsiness, constipation and dry mouth.

In recent years, new antiemetic molecules have been developed, offering greater efficacy and fewer side effects. Combination therapies, which combine different antiemetics such as corticosteroids and 5-HT3 receptor antagonists, have shown promising clinical results. In addition, emerging technologies such as transdermal devices and sustained-release systems are improving adherence to treatment while side effects.

12. References

1. Zhong W, Shahbaz O, Teskey G, Beever A, Kachour N, Venketaraman V, Darmani NA. Mechanisms of Nausea and Vomiting: Current Knowledge and Recent Advances in Intracellular Emetic Signaling Systems. International Journal of Molecular Sciences, 22(11), 5797; 2021 [**Online**]. Available on : Sci-Hub | Mechanisms of Nausea and Vomiting: Current Knowledge and Recent Advances in Intracellular Emetic Signaling Systems. International Journal of Molecular Sciences, 22(11), 5797 | 10.3390/ijms22115797 (Consulted on 01/05/2023).
2. Denholm, L., & Gallagher, G. (2021). Physiology and pharmacology of nausea and vomiting. Anaesthesia & Intensive Care Medicine. Available on: Sci-Hub | Physiology and pharmacology of nausea and vomiting. Anaesthesia & Intensive Care Medicine | 10.1016/j.mpaic.2021.07.002 (Consulted on 01 /05/2023).
3. Sanger, G. J., & Andrews, P. L. R. (2018). A History of Drug Discovery for Treatment of Nausea and Vomiting and the Implications for Future Research. Frontiers in Pharmacology, 9.[Online]. Available from: Sci-Hub | A History of Drug Discovery for Treatment of Nausea and Vomiting and the Implications for Future Research. Frontiers in Pharmacology, 9 | 10.3389/fphar.2018.00913 (Accessed 01/05/2023).
4. Athavale A, Athavale T, Roberts DM. Antiemetic drugs: what to prescribe and when. Aust Prescr. 2020 Apr;43(2):49-56 [**Online**]. Available from: Antiemetic drugs: what to prescribe and when - PMC (nih.gov) (Accessed 01 /05/2023).
5. Gale, J. D., & Mori, I. (2007). Emesis/Prokinetic Agents. Comprehensive Medicinal Chemistry II, 671-691 [**On line**]. Available on: Sci-Hub | Emesis/Prokinetic Agents. Comprehensive Medicinal Chemistry II, 671-691 | 10.1016/b0-08-045044-x/00191-KConsulted 01/05/2023).
6. Isola S, Hussain A, Dua A, et al. Metoclopramide. In: StatPearls. Treasure Island (FL): StatPearls Publishing; 2023. [**On-line**]. Available from: https://www.ncbi.nlm.nih.gov/books/NBK519517/ (Accessed 01/05/2023).
7. European Directorate for the Quality of Medicines and Healthcare. Metoclopramide

monograph. **In**: *European Pharmacopoeia*. 9th ed. France: EDQM, 2018, p. 3272-3273.
8. European Directorate for the Quality of Medicines and Healthcare. Ondansetron product monograph. **In**: *European Pharmacopoeia*. 9th ed. France: EDQM, 2018, p. 3438-3439.
9. European Directorate for the Quality of Medicines and Healthcare. Aprepitant product monograph. **In**: *European Pharmacopoeia*. 9th ed. France: EDQM, 2018, p. 1881-1882.

Chapter 2

Antispasmodic medicines

1. Introduction

Antispasmodics are an essential therapeutic class, used to alleviate painful involuntary muscle spasms, particularly in the gastrointestinal tract. These spasms can be triggered by a variety of pathophysiological factors. The excessive smooth muscle contraction that characterises these spasms often results from dysregulation of the neuronal receptors or intracellular mechanisms involved in muscle contractility. Antispasmodics act primarily by modulating these pathophysiological mechanisms.

2. A reminder of the physiology of intestinal motricity

The gastrointestinal tract (GI tract) is made up hollow organs including the resophagus, stomach, small intestine and colon, which are themselves made up two layers of muscle: a longitudinal outer layer and a circular inner layer. It is also made up sphincters. These are contracted at rest. These are: the upper resophageal sphincter (SSO), the lower resophageal sphincter (SIO), the pyloric sphincter, the ileocecal valve and the anal sphincter (internal and external).

The organs that make up the gastrointestinal tract are surrounded by specific muscles that allow their walls to contract in order perform certain functions. The muscles are initially striated, with the tongue, pharynx and upper 1/3 of the resophagus, then become smooth up to the anal sphincter (note that the latter is striated).

In most cases, motor skills are not dependent on willpower.

The striated muscles (a minority in the TD) are dependent on willpower for swallowing and defecation. But the smooth muscles (the majority), which depend on the autonomic nervous system (ANS), do not, and are therefore independent of the will. This is said to be a matter of reflex.

2.1. Different types of contractions

There are different types of contractions:

> They can be in the form of localised pinching (of little use for the spread of the alimentary bolus), or segmentation movements: pinching of 2 adjacent segments but has disadvantages.

> Or they may be of the propagated type (often anterograde). These contractions are responsible for peristalsis in the gastrointestinal tract, as they serve to move food along the tract when they become phasic. In fact, phasic propagated contractions are carried out periodically, moving from the stomach to the colon via the circular and longitudinal muscle layers.

The digestive system, in association with the action of the muscles, serves a number of functions, such as: the progression of the bolus of food to enable it to be transported along the tube, digestion, with the mixing of food, secretions/excretions and absorption. It also acts as a reservoir (stomach, colon ++).

Smooth muscle cells alone are incapable of producing the motor activity of the digestive tract. Their contractile activity is initiated by the action of Cajal's interstitial cells (CICs), mainly located between the two muscle layers. The CICs also control motor activity in association with the intrinsic nervous system, located in the wall of the digestive tract.

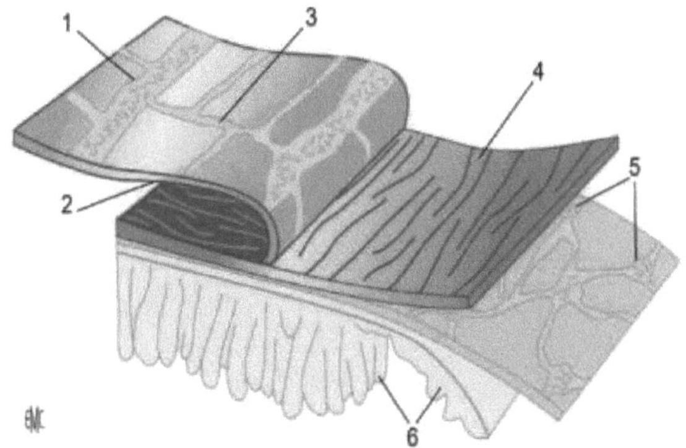

Figure 1: Structure of digestive smooth muscle (Roman et al, 2009).

2.2. Contractile activity of the digestive tract: role of smooth muscle cells

Muscle fibres are organised into bundles a dozen or so cells, called contractile units. They are joined together in a functional syncytium. All the cells forming the same syncytium relax and contract at the same time. The orientation of the muscle cells depends on the layer in which they are located: it is longitudinal in the longitudinal layer and transverse in the circular layer.

Smooth muscle contraction and relaxation are based on the interaction of actin and myosin filaments present in the cytoplasm of muscle cells. Their occurrence depends on the phosphorylation of myosin. This is regulated by two enzymes: a specific kinase, myosin light chain kinase (MLCK), and a specific phosphatase (myosin light chain phosphatase [MLCP]).

The calcium-calmodulin complex that is formed activates an enzyme, myosin light chain kinase. This kinase enables the phosphorylation of one of the two light myosin chains on each myosin head using ATP. This phosphorylation unmasks the actin binding site on the heavy myosin head. The binding of actin to myosin induces contraction of the smooth muscle fibre.

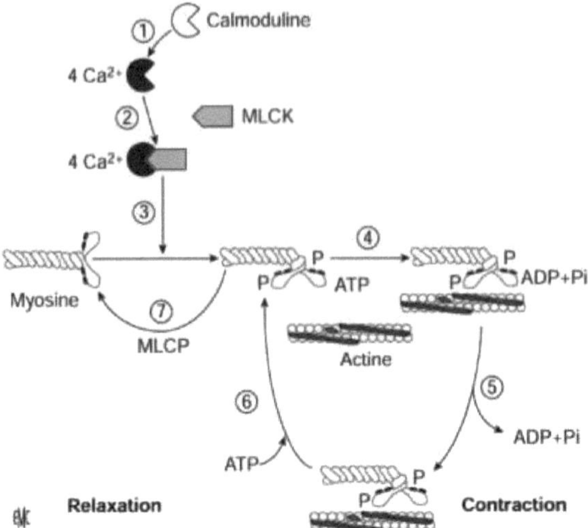

Figure 2: Interaction of contractile proteins during smooth muscle contraction and relaxation (Roman et al, 2009).

2.3. Automatism and synchronisation of motor activity: role of Cajal's interstitial cells

Cajal's interstitial cells are responsible for the automatism of the digestive tract (pacemaker role) and the synchronisation of motor activity. They play an essential role in linking motor neurons (excitatory or inhibitory) and smooth muscle cells. In certain areas, the CICs are grouped together to form veritable local pacemakers, for example in the gastric body at the level of the greater curvature. On the other hand, they are distributed along the entire length of the small intestine and colon. The absence of Cajal's cells is the cause of various digestive motor disorders such achalasia and Hirschsprung's disease.

2.4. Spontaneous activity of digestive smooth muscle

The major difference between striated muscle and smooth muscle is that smooth muscle is endowed with automatism, whereas the motor activity of striated muscle is subordinate to control by the extrinsic nervous system. For example, an isolated segment of intestine placed in a survival fluid contracts regularly. This intestinal motor activity depends on the occurrence slow waves. These are generated by Cajal's cells and propagate to the smooth muscle cells throughout the digestive tract. The action potentials of the muscle cells are responsible for the occurrence of mechanical activity.

2.4.1. Spontaneous electrical activity of Cajal cells

The spontaneous electrical activity of Cajal's cells is initiated by the intracytoplasmic release of calcium via the activity of IP3 receptors present on the membrane of the endoplasmic reticulum. Calcium activates chlorine channels on the plasma membrane. Chlorine movements induce variations in the membrane potential, known as the unit potential. According to other authors, the calcium released into the intracellular space is recaptured by the mitochondria located close to the endoplasmic reticulum. This decrease in intracytoplasmic calcium activates the non-selective conductance of the plasma membrane to cations and thus induces variations in the membrane potential , the unit potentials. The summation of different unit potentials opens the voltage-dependent calcium channels present on the plasma membrane and creates a depolarisation current. The depolarisation is transmitted from one Cajal's cell to another via the communicating junctions. The activation of voltage-gated calcium channels in the second Cajal cell by the depolarisation current is responsible for an influx of calcium into the intracellular medium. This increases the sensitivity of IP3 receptors on the endoplasmic reticulum membrane and promotes the release of calcium into the cytoplasm.

2.4.2. Coordination of motor activity by the nervous system

Neuroendocrine regulation plays a role in coordinating muscular activity to ensure the mixing and propulsion of the alimentary bolus from the resophagus to the anus. The wall of the digestive tract is very rich in neurons.

There is a majority of intrinsic (or enteric) innervation, located entirely in the digestive wall, and extrinsic innervation, the neurons of which have cell bodies outside the digestive wall.

> **. Intrinsic innervation**

Different types of neuron make up the intrinsic nervous system.

> **Sensory neurons**

Intrinsic primary afferent neurons (IPANs) play a role in detecting mechanical and chemical stimuli. They are located in the submucosa and between the two muscle layers.

The main neurotransmitters involved are acetylcholine, substance P and tachykinins. The release of serotonin by digestive endocrine cells is responsible for activating these neurons.

> **Motor neurons**

The motor neurons of the enteric nervous system are divided into ganglionic clusters and form two main plexuses:

> **The myenteric plexus**, located between the two muscle layers (Auerbach's plexus), is responsible for motor control;

> **The submucosal plexus** in the submucosa (Meissner's plexus) is involved in controlling gastrointestinal secretions and local blood flow.

In addition, the plexuses receive afferents from the extrinsic nervous system (sympathetic and parasympathetic) and emit primary efferent axons that ascend to the central nervous system.

The axons of the motor neurons of the enteric nervous system do not have a synapse at the end but have varicosities along their entire length. These varicosities allow direct projection of the motor neurons onto the smooth muscle cells of the longitudinal layer or the circular layer, but also onto Cajal's cells. Activation of the two muscle layers by the enteric system is independent of each other.

Some neurons stimulate the contraction of smooth muscle cells, while others inhibit it. Excitatory motor neurons predominate in the digestive tract (with the exception of the lower sphincter of the resophagus). Their main mediators acetylcholine, substance P and tachykinins. By stimulating them, the amplitude of the slow waves rises above a sufficient threshold to generate calcium-dependent membrane potentials that cause the smooth muscle cells to contract.

Inhibitory motor neurons are mediated by vaso intestinal peptide and nitric oxide (NO). Their activation blocks the contractile muscle response by inhibiting calcium action .

2.5. Digestive motor pathologies

2.5.1. Esophageal spasm

In this condition, the normal peristaltic contractions that propel food through the resophagus are periodically replaced by non-propulsive contractions or excessive muscular contractions (hyperdynamia) that do not move food through the resophagus.

The exact cause of this condition is not known and symptoms include chest pain below the breastbone and difficulty swallowing.

2.5.2. Abdominal spasm

These are **involuntary contractions of the abdominal digestive muscles**. These muscles are not under the individual's voluntary control and function automatically to peristalsis, which allows the digestive contents to move forward. "**Abdominal spasms occur in the form of attacks responsible for pain or a feeling of discomfort** that can last from a few seconds to several hours, or even several days. Abdominal pain can be characterised by its **recurrent** nature (referred to as chronic abdominal pain) **or by its one-off** nature (referred to as acute abdominal pain)".

These spasms may also be **accompanied by other symptoms such as nausea, vomiting or transit disorders**. They may be related to an abdominal pathology, but may also occur spontaneously, without any obvious cause.

> Abdominal spasm on the left side

They can indicate :

- Intestinal problems such as **constipation** or **gas** formation.
- **Irritable bowel syndrome.**
- Muscle spasms (side stitches).
- Spleen or kidney damage.

> Abdominal spasm on the right side

They can indicate :

- Liver damage.
- Intestinal damage.
- Appendicitis.

> Abdominal spasms in the subumbilical region

They can be a sign of :

- A urinary infection.
- Damage to the ovaries or fallopian tubes.

3. History of discovery and development

Antispasmodics have been discovered and developed over the decades to meet a variety of medical needs. Their history dates back to ancient times, when plants were used to treat abdominal pain and cramps. The use of plants such as peppermint and chamomile has been documented in ancient Egypt, Greece and Rome.

The first antispasmodics were discovered in the nineteenth century. In 1838, Dr Formby of Liverpool was the first to use chloroform as an antispasmodic tranquilliser. In 1842, Dr Mortimer Glover, a young doctor from Edinburgh, discovered through his experiments that chloroform was a very powerful narcotic poison.

Belladonna was first isolated in the 19th century. Belladonna, also known as Atropa belladona, is a poisonous plant that was used in the era to dilate the pupils. Later, belladonna's antispasmodic properties were discovered and used to treat muscle spasms in the stomach and intestine.

In the early 20th century, antispasmodics derived from belladonna, such as hyoscine, were developed to treat muscle spasms in the stomach and intestine. During the Second World War, antispasmodics were used to relieve the symptoms of mustard gas poisoning, which causes muscle spasms.

In the 1950s, the first synthetic antispasmodics, such as PAPAVERINE and DROTAVERINE, were developed. These drugs have a similar structure to atropine, but are less toxic and have more specific effects on the digestive system.

Over the years, antispasmodics have been developed to treat different types of muscle spasm. PHLOROGLUCINOL is a musculotropic antispasmodic belonging to the triphenol family1. It was discovered by Gérard Glauert and Jacques Fleuret in 1890, CLIDINIUM in 1950, TRIMEBUTINE, PINAVERIUM, MEBEVERINE in 1960 and OXYBUTININE in 1970.

4. Classification of antispasmodics

Antispasmodics are used to treat spasmodic and painful symptoms in the digestive and urinary tracts, as well as in gynaecology and obstetrics.
There are two types of antispasmodics:

- **Anticholingergic antispasmodics ;**
- **Musculotropic antispasmodics.**

Their difference lies in their **mode of action**. The former act by blocking the receptors for acetylcholine, a neurotransmitter that plays a role in muscle activity, while the latter act directly on the muscles to relieve spasms".

5. Anticholinergic antispasmodics

Anticholinergic antispasmodics act on neurotransmitters. They stop the action of acetylcholine on synapses. This inhibition blocks the arrival of nerve impulses. In this way, the muscles are no longer dependent on the parasympathetic system, causing them to relax (Table I).
Atropine is the parent substance of anticholinergics. It is capable of antagonising the muscarinic effects of acetylcholine. It therefore inhibits most of the effects of excitation of the parasympathetic system.
Derivatives have been synthesised obtain a more specific spasmolytic or anti-secretory response. There are ester derivatives with a tertiary amine group and ester derivatives with a quaternary amine group (including Buscopan®, hyoscine butylbromide).

Table I. Main anticholinergic antispasmodics.

Molecule INN	Trade name and pharmaceutical form	Chemical structure and scientific name
Atropine	***ATNAA®, ATROPEN®, BUSULFEX®*** Solution injectable : 1 mg/mL Collyre : 0,5% (5 mg/mL)	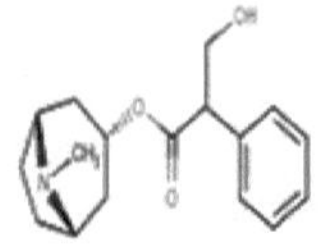 (1R,3r,5S,7S,8S)-8-(hydroxyméthyl)-3-[(1R,2R,4S)-2-hydroxy-4-{[(2S,3R,4S,5S,6R)-3,4,5-trihydroxy-6-(hydroxyméthyl)oxan-2-yl]oxy}-1-méthylpentoxy]-8-méthyl-8-azoniabicyclo[3.2.1]octane
Bromure de N-butylhyocyamine	***BUSCOPAN®*** Comprimés : 10 mg Solution injectable : 20 mg/1 mL	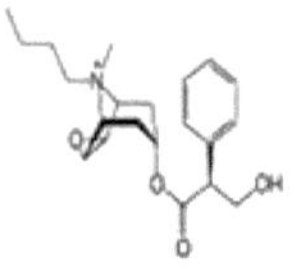 Bromure de N-butylhyoscyamine

Table I. Main anticholinergic antispasmodics (continued).

Molecule INN	Trade name and pharmaceutical form	Chemical structure and scientific name
Clidinium	***LIBRAX®*** (en association à un neuroleptique : chlordiaéepoxide)	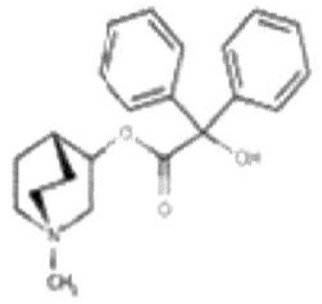 3-benzhydrylquinuclidine-3-car boxylate de 2-bromobenzyle
Oxybutinine	***DITROPAN®*** Comprimés à libération prolongée à 5 mg	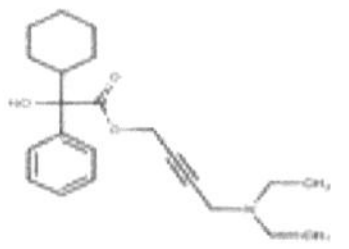 (RS)-N-(4-diéthylaminoéthyl)-3-hydroxy-2-phenyl-propanamide
Prifinium	***RIABAL®*** Comprimés pelliculés à 10 mg	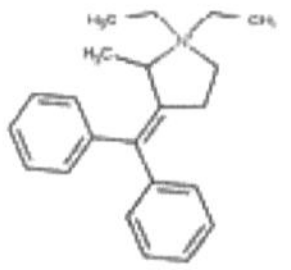 (RS)-1-[2-(4-chlorophényl)-2-hydroxyéthyl]-1,2,3,4-tétra hydro-6,7-diméthoxy-2-mét hylisoquinoline
Tiemonium	***VISCERALGINE®*** Solution buvable	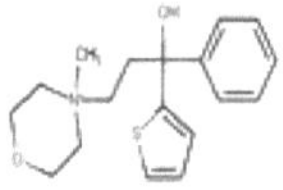 (RS)-3-[(2-hydroxy-2,2-diphény léthyl)diméthylammonio]propan oate

5.1. Lead study

Atropine: *ATROPEN®*

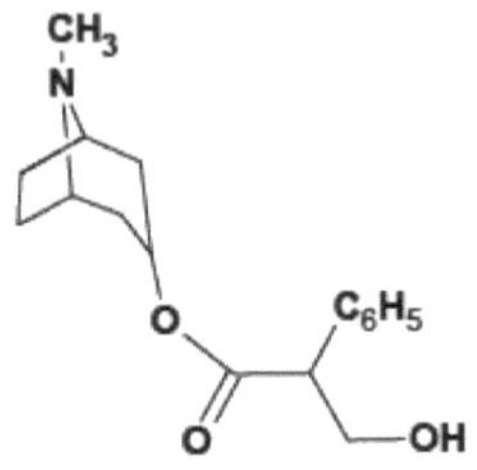

Figure 3: Chemical structure of atropine.

5.1.1. Chemical synthesis

It can be synthesised using a standard tropane alkaloid synthesis scheme.

The condensation of maleylaldehyde with methylamine and 3-ketonedicarboxylic acid gives tropenone, which is the main raw material for the synthesis of atropine and scopolamine.

The carbonyl group of tropenone is reduced, forming tropenol, and the double bond between C6 and C7 of the tropane ring is then hydrogenated, giving tropine. Esterification of tropenol gives atropine.

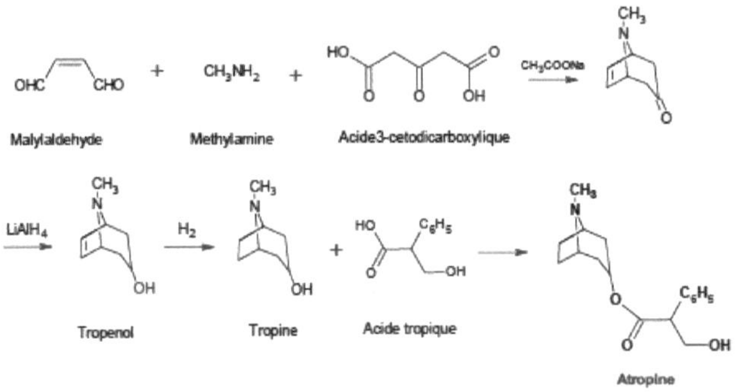

Figure 4: Chemical synthesis of atropine.

5.1.2. Analytical control

1. Physico-chemical properties

Atropine is a white or almost white crystalline powder or colourless crystals. Very soluble in water, easily soluble in ethanol.

2. Identification

- Optical rotation angle
- Infrared absorption spectrophotometry
- Atropine sulphate gives sulphate reactions
- Atropine sulphate gives the alkaloid reaction

3. Test

— PH

— Optical rotation angle: - 0.50° to + 0.05°.

— Related substances

- Water

- Sulphuric ash

4. Dosage

Titration by potentiometry.

5.2. Structure-activity relationship

Anticholinergic compounds can be considered as chemicals that have a certain similarity to ACh, but which also contain substituents that reinforce their binding to the cholinergic receptor.

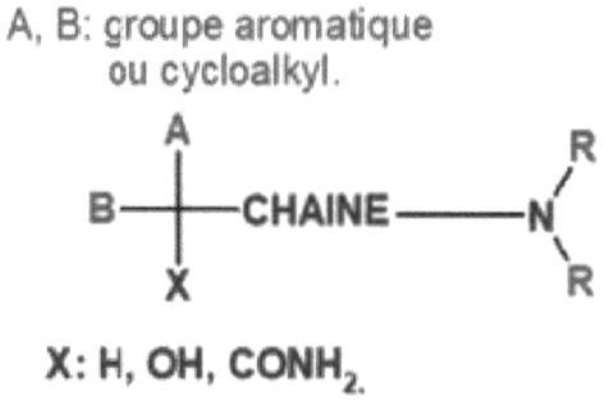

A, B: groupe aromatique
ou cycloalkyl.

A
B—CHAINE——N(R)(R)
X

X: H, OH, $CONH_2$.

Figure 5. Common structure of anticholinergics.

> **The cationic head**

Anticholinergic molecules are generally considered to have a primary attachment point at the cholinergic site via the cationic head (i.e. the positively charged nitrogen).

For quaternary ammonium compounds, there is no doubt about what this implies, but for tertiary amines, it is correctly assumed that the cationic head is obtained by protonation of the amine at physiological pH.

N-linked alkyl groups (R) can be superior to methyl (as opposed to agonists). When N1 groups are ethyl or isopropyl, the effect is maximised but toxicity is increased.

Quaternary N can be found in the ring (pyridine, piperidine, pyrrolidine). While agonists must carry a quarternary nitrogen, the antagonist nitrogen can be tertiary or quaternary. It should be noted, however, that the tertiary nitrogen atom is charged when it interacts with the receptor.

> **Substitution of the carbon in position a**

A suitably placed alcoholic hydroxyl group antimuscarinic activity compared to a similar compound without a hydroxyl group. The position of the hydroxyl group relative to the nitrogen appears to be quite critical, with the diameter of the receptive zone estimated to be around 2 to 3 Angstroms. It is assumed that the hydroxyl group contributes to the strength of the bond, probably by hydrogen bonding to an electron-rich part of the receptor surface.

> The hydroxy group or the hydroxy-methyl group is the most potent antagonist.

> R 2 and R3 must be carboxylic or heterocyclic rings (phenyl, cyclohexyl, cyclopentyl) for maximum antagonistic power.

> Substitution of the naphthalene rings at R2 and R3 results in inactive compounds due to steric hindrance at the muscarinic receptor.

> Larger R2 and R3 groups bind to the outer hydrophobic region of the acetylcholine receptor.

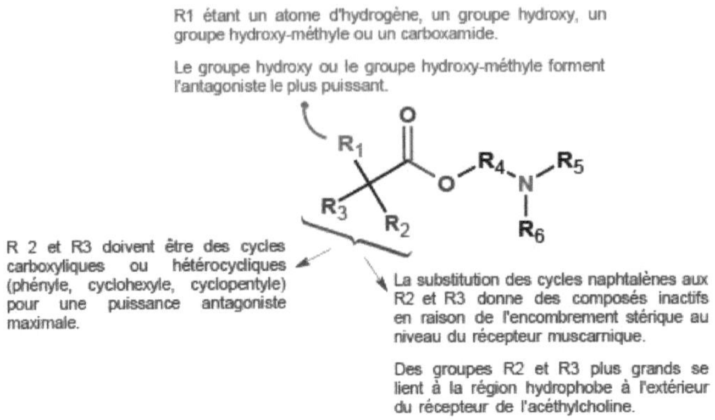

R1 étant un atome d'hydrogène, un groupe hydroxy, un groupe hydroxy-méthyle ou un carboxamide.

Le groupe hydroxy ou le groupe hydroxy-méthyle forment l'antagoniste le plus puissant.

R 2 et R3 doivent être des cycles carboxyliques ou hétérocycliques (phényle, cyclohexyle, cyclopentyle) pour une puissance antagoniste maximale.

La substitution des cycles naphtalènes aux R2 et R3 donne des composés inactifs en raison de l'encombrement stérique au niveau du récepteur muscarnique.

Des groupes R2 et R3 plus grands se lient à la région hydrophobe à l'extérieur du récepteur de l'acéthylcholine.

R1 being a hydrogen , a hydroxy group, a hydroxy-methyl group or a carboxamide.
The hydroxy or hydroxy-methyl group is the most powerful antagonist.

R 2 and R3 must be carboxylic or heterocyclic rings (phenyl, cyclohexyl, cyclopentyl) for maximum antagonistic potency.
R2 and R3 give inactive compounds due to steric hindrance at the muscarinic receptor.

Larger R2 and R3 groups bind to the hydrophobic region on the outside of the acetylcholine receptor.

Figure 6. Structural changes to the carbon in position a.

The ester group

Many very potent antimuscarinic compounds have an ester group, which can contribute to effective binding. This is reasonable because the agonist has a similar function or binds to the same site.

An ester function is not necessary for the activity, as several types of compound do not have such a group (e.g. ethers, aminoalcohols).

the ester group may also be also an ether, or be totally absent	the ester group provides anticholinergic activity

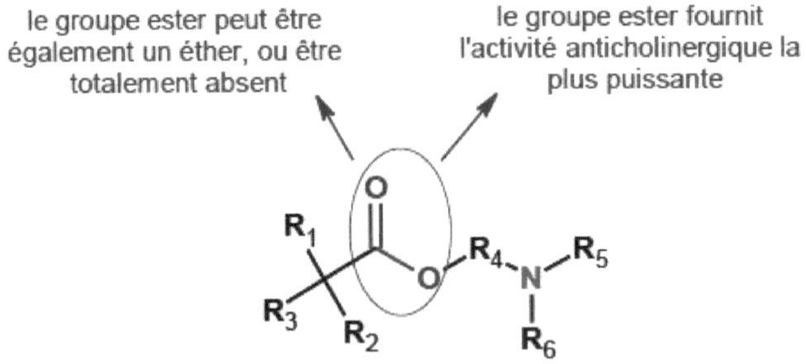

le groupe ester peut être également un éther, ou être totalement absent

le groupe ester fournit l'activité anticholinergique la plus puissante

Figure 7. Structural changes to the ester group.

> Cyclic substitution

Active compounds have at least one cyclic substituent (phenyl, thienyl or other), a feature common to almost all anticholinergic molecules. Aromatic substitution is often used in connection with the acidic part of the ester function.

Large acids {Mandelic, Tropic, Benzilik, etc.} are necessary for activity. (Very large acyl groups can be present (A and B = aromatic or heteroaromatic ring), unlike agonists for which only acetyl groups are acceptable).

5.3. Mechanism of action

Anticholinergic antispasmodic agents are a class of drugs used to treat a variety of conditions involving muscle contraction and relaxation, including gastrointestinal cramps, muscle spasms and diarrhoea.
Anticholinergics block the action of acetylcholine (a chemical messenger) released by the nerves to cause muscle contraction.
Blocking acetylcholine inhibits involuntary muscle movements and various other bodily functions. Antispasmodics slow down the natural movements of the intestine and help to relax the stomach and intestinal muscles.
Anticholinergic antispasmodics block action of a neurotransmitter called acetylcholine in the central and peripheral nervous systems.
Acetylcholine is responsible for transferring signals between certain cells that carry out specific bodily functions (notably digestion, micturition and salivation).
They prevent acetylcholine from binding to its receptors on certain nerve cells, which inhibits involuntary muscle movements in the lungs, gastrointestinal tract, urinary tract and other parts of the body.
Anticholinergic agents reduce the production of acid in the stomach, which slows down the natural movements of the intestine, thus relaxing the muscles of numerous organs such as the stomach, intestines, kidneys and bladder. They also reduce the quantity of body fluids (saliva, sweat).

5.4. Indications

Anticholinergic antispasmodic agents are used to treat the following:
> Gastrointestinal disorders
— Peptic ulcer (wounds that develop in the lining of the stomach, lower resophagus or small intestine)
— Irritable bowel syndrome (intestinal disorder causing stomach pain, diarrhoea and constipation)
— Abdominal cramps
- Diverticulitis (small bulging pouches that can form in the lining of the digestive system)
- Diarrhoea
> **Cramps caused by**
- Kidney stones
- Gallstones
> **Preoperative medication for :**
- Promoting relaxation
- Controlling heart rate
- Reduce salivation
> Overactive bladder (frequent and sudden urge urinate which can be difficult to control)
> Parkinson's disease (a brain disorder that causes tremors, stiffness and difficulty with walking, balance and coordination)
> Sialorrhoea (excessive drooling or salivation - a common problem in children with neurological disorders)
> Pylorospasm (spasm of the pyloric sphincter often accompanied by pain and vomiting).

5.5. Side effects

Atropine derivatives or anticholinergic antispasmodics are used less frequently because of the frequency of side effects. These anticholinergics inhibit the effects of stimulation of the parasympathetic system by acting on the receptors and, as a result, inhibit the effects of

acetylcholine, which can lead to side effects.
In fact, their use can be accompanied by two types of side-effect, either peripheral or central.
> **The peripheral effects** are: tachycardia, dry mouth, hyperthermia (rise in body temperature) due to inhibition of sweating, reddening of the skin (dilation of skin vessels to promote heat release by increasing cutaneous blood flow to compensate for the hyperthermia) and constipation (due to blockage of intestinal peristalsis).
> **Central effects** include motor agitation, hallucinations and confusion.

6. Musculotropic antispasmodics

They act directly on the smooth muscle fibres (to encourage them to relax and relieve the spasm) and not on the neuromediator.
They act on the smooth muscle fibres of the digestive tract, urinary tract and uterine muscle.
They are indicated in particular for hepatic and nephritic colic, spasmodic and painful symptoms, and the biliary, urinary and uterine tracts, and have fewer side-effects than anticholinergic antispasmodics.
The parent substance of this family is **PAPAVERINE**. It is an alkaloid extracted from papaver somniferum. It interferes with smooth muscle contraction by inhibiting the transmembrane transfer of $Ca^{(2+)}$ ions. It has a predominant effect on the peripheral and cerebral vascular system. It causes vasodilatation.
The basic structure of PAPAVERINE is used to synthesise products with a more selective musculotropic spasmolytic action on digestive, urological and gynaecological smooth fibres.
One of these derivatives is PHLOROGLUCINOL: ***SPASFON®*** (table II).

Table II. Main musculotropic antispasmodics.

Molecule INN	Trade name and pharmaceutical form	Chemical structure and scientific name
Papavérine	***PAPAVERINE®*** Comprimés 40 mg, 80 mg	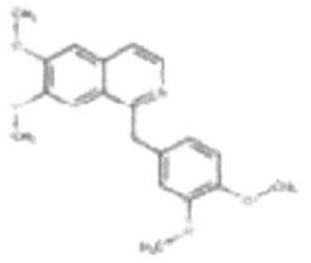 (RS)-1-[(3,4-diméthoxyphényl) mét hyl]-6,7-diméthoxyisoquinoline
Chlorhydrate de mébévérine	***COLPRONE®*** Comprimés : 200 mg	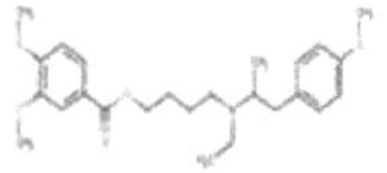 N,N-diméthyl-2-[(1-méthoxy prop an-2-yl)amino]éthyl 2-(4-méthoxy phényl)acétate
Citrate d'Alvérine	***SPASMODEX®*** Comprimés : 60 mg	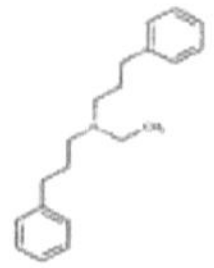 acide (RS)-2-[(4-éthoxyphényl) méthyl]-2,3-dihydro-1H-indole-6-carboxylate de 1-méthyl pipé razine
Maléate de Trimébutine	***DEBRIDAT®*** Comprimés : 100 mg 200mg	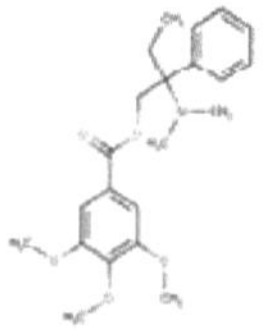 (RS)-2-(diéthylamino)éthyl (3,4,5-triméthoxybenzoate) méthylamine

Table II. Main musculotropic antispasmodics (continued).

Molecule INN	Trade name and pharmaceutical form	Chemical structure and scientific name
Phloroglucinol	***SPASFON®*** Comprimés lyophilisés à 80 mg et 160 mg	1,3,5-trihydroxybenzène
Pinavérium	***DICETEL®*** Comprimés pelliculés à50 mg et 100 mg	(RS)-1-(4-éthoxybenzyl)-6,7-di méthoxy-1,2,3,4-tétrahydroiso quinoline

6.2. Study of the lead partner

Phloroglucinol*: SPASFON®* (in French)

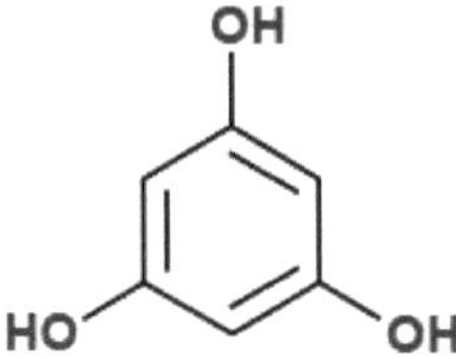

Figure 8. Chemical structure of Phloroglucinol.

Phloroglucinol or benzene-1,3,5-triol is a musculotropic antispasmodic. It was discovered by Gérard Glauert and Jacques Fleuret.

It is frequently prescribed relieve spasms in functional digestive disorders (colitis), renal or hepatic colic and certain gynaecological complaints.

6.2.1. Chemical synthesis

It can be synthesised in a number of ways, one of the most representative being from trinitrobenzene.

Figure 9. Chemical synthesis of Phloroglucinol.

6.2.2. Quality control

1. Physico-chemical properties

Phloroglucinol is a white or approximately white powder. It is fairly soluble in water, easily soluble in 96% ethanol and practically insoluble in methylene chloride.

2. Identification

- Infrared absorption spectrophotometry
- Thin layer chromatography

3. Test

- Assay of related substances by liquid chromatography.
- Test for loss on drying, heavy metals and sulphuric ash.

4. Dosage

Titration by potentiometry.

1.3. Mechanism of action

Musculotropic antispasmodic drugs, such as DICYCLOMINE and MEBEVERINE, belong to the class of drugs known as **calcium channel blockers**. These drugs act by blocking the influx calcium ions through voltage-gated L-type calcium channels in smooth muscle cells.

Musculotropic antispasmodic drugs bind to specific sites on **L-type calcium channels**, preventing calcium ions from entering the cells. The result is a decrease in intracellular calcium concentration, leading to relaxation of smooth muscle cells and relief of spasms.

In addition to their effects on calcium channels, musculotropic antispasmodic drugs can also have effects on other ion channels, such as potassium channels. By increasing efflux of potassium ions from smooth muscle cells, these drugs can enhance smooth muscle relaxation.

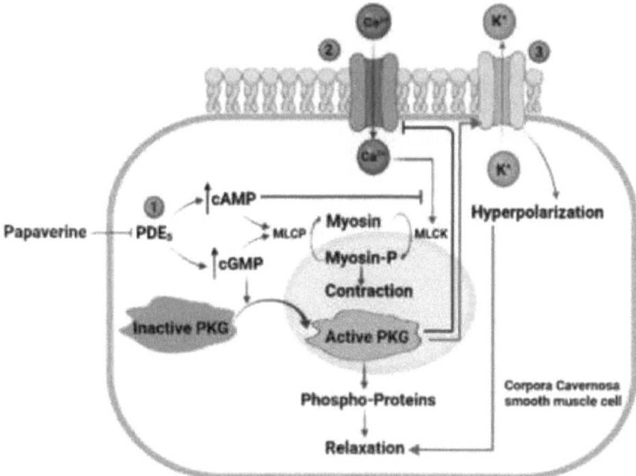

Figure 10. Mechanism of action of Papaverine.

1.4. Indications

Musculotropic antispasmodics are used to treat various disorders characterised by smooth muscle spasms. Here are some common indications for these drugs:

- Irritable bowel syndrome (IBS).
- Biliary colic.
- Renal colic.
- Biliary dyskinesia.
- Menstrual pain (dysmenorrhoea).

- Diverticulitis.
- Spasmodic colitis.
- Intestinal colic.

Musculotropic antispasmodics act directly on smooth muscle to reduce spasm without affecting normal bowel motility, making them useful in a variety of gastrointestinal and urological conditions where muscle spasm is a major problem.

1.5. Undesirable effects

Adverse reactions to direct muscle relaxants are very rare. When they are reported, the most common side effects are as follows:

- Dry mouth.
- Nausea.
- Dizziness.
- Indigestion.
- Heartburn.
- Constipation.
- Insomnia (sleep disorders).
- Anorexia (loss appetite or refusal eat).
- Headaches.
- Fatigue.
- Unusual muscle movements.
- Skin rash or itching.

7. Conclusion and outlook

Antispasmodics are indispensable therapeutic agents in the management of smooth muscle spasms, which are a common feature of many gastrointestinal, urological and gynaecological conditions. By acting on various pathophysiological mechanisms, in particular by modulating the activity of muscarinic receptors, inhibiting the enzymes responsible for muscle contractility, or modifying neuronal transmission, antispasmodics effectively relieve painful symptoms and improve patients' quality of life.

The outlook for antispasmodics is varied and promising. Advances in the development of new agents, the optimisation of current therapies, personalised approaches and the integration of non-pharmacological therapies are opening up new avenues for improving the management of muscle spasms. These concerted efforts aim to offer therapeutic solutions that are more effective, safer and tailored to individual patient needs, thereby contributing to a better quality of life for those suffering from these conditions.

8. References

1. Roman, S., & Mion, F. (2009). Fundamental data on the physiology of digestive motricity. EMC - Gastro-Enterology, 4(4), 1-8. [Available on: Données fondamentales sur la Physiologie de la motricité digestive - EM consulte (em-consulte.com).
2. Ouyang A, Locke GR: Overview of neurogastroenterology- gastrointestinal motility and function GI disorders: classification, prevalence, and epidemiology. Gastroenterol Clin North Am 36:485 498, 2007.
3. SeowCY.Myosinfilamentassemblyinanever-changingmyofilament lattice of smooth muscle. Am J Physiol Cell Physiol 2005;289: C1363C1368.
4. Harnett KM, Cao W, Biancani P. Signal-transduction pathways that regulate smooth muscle function I. Signal transduction in phasic (esophageal) and tonic (gastroesophageal sphincter) smooth muscles. AmJPhysiol Gastrointest Liver Physiol 2005;288:G407-G416.
5. Khandekar Hussan Reza et al. Mechanism of action of cholinergic drugs. Academic Press,2023. ISBN 9780323998550.p.27-46. [Available at : Mechanism of action of

cholinergic drugs - ScienceDirect.
6. Szymaszkiewicz, A., & Zieliñska, M. (2020). Irritable bowel syndrome: Current therapies and future perspectives. A Comprehensive Overview of Irritable Bowel Syndrome, 129-144 [On line] Available at : Irritable bowel syndrome: Current therapies and future perspectives - ScienceDirect.
7. Hicks, G. A. (2007). Irritable Bowel Syndrome. Comprehensive Medicinal Chemistry II, 643-670 [On line] Available at : Irritable Bowel Syndrome - ScienceDirect.
8. Videlock EJ, Chang L: Irritable bowel syndrome-current approach to symptoms, evaluation, and treatment. Gastroenterol Clin North Am 36:665-685, 2007.
9. Washabau, R. J. (2013). Antispasmodic Agents. Canine and Feline Gastroenterology, 481-485. *[*Available at : Antispasmodic Agents - ScienceDirect.
10. European Directorate for the Quality of Medicines and Healthcare. Atropine monograph. **In**: *European Pharmacopoeia*. 9th ed. France: EDQM, 2018, p. 1915-1916.
11. European Directorate for the Quality of Medicines and Healthcare. Phloroglucinol monograph. **In**: *European Pharmacopoeia*. 9th ed. France: EDQM, 2018, p. 3556-3557.

Chapter 3

Medicines for Gastric Acidity

1. Introduction

Gastric acidity is a normal physiological phenomenon, necessary for the digestion of food and protection against infection. However, excessive production of gastric acid can lead to various gastrointestinal disorders, such as gastro- resophageal reflux disease (GERD), gastric and duodenal ulcers and dyspepsia.

Anti-gastric acid drugs, or antisecretory drugs, are essential in the management and treatment of these conditions. They act primarily by reducing the production of hydrochloric acid by the stomach, neutralising acid already present or protecting the gastric mucosa from the corrosive effects of acid.

2. Pathophysiological background

2.1. Anatomy of the stomach

The stomach is located between the resophagus and the duodenum, in the epigastric, umbilical and left hypochondrium regions of the abdomen. It is the most dilated part of the gastrointestinal tract and is subdivided into four regions:

- The cardia, which surrounds the opening of the resophagus into the stomach;
- The gastric fundus, which is the area above the orifice of the cardia ;
- The body of the stomach, the largest region, is the middle section, which extends downwards into the funnel-shaped pyloric section;
- The pyloric portion, which is the distal portion of the stomach and is divided into the pyloric antrum and the pyloric duct.
- The greater curvature, where the gastrosplenic ligament and greater omentum are inserted;
- The lesser curvature, where the lesser omentum is inserted;
- The cardiac incisure, which is the upper angle created by the penetration of the resophagus into the stomach;
- The angular incisure, which is an inflection in the minor curvature (Figure 1).

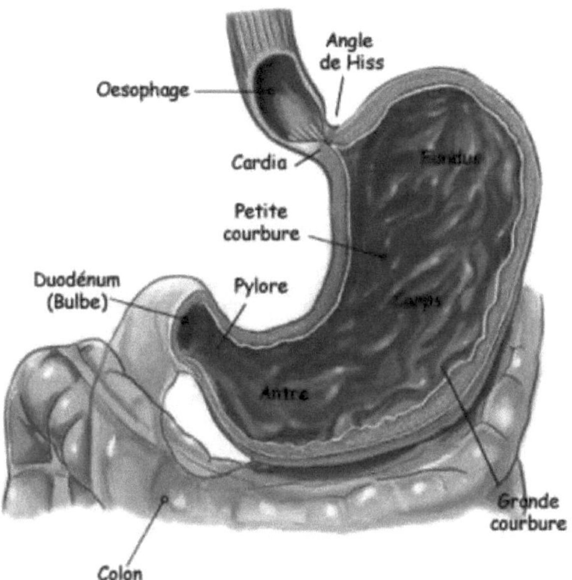

Figure 1. Anatomy of the stomach (Mennecier; 2022).

2.2. Histology of the stomach

The stomach lining is made up of four layers:

- An internal mucosa when the stomach is empty it forms large folds, called gastric folds, the surface of the mucosa is a layer of simple prismatic non-ciliated epithelial cells called superficial mucus cells;
- A submucosa with numerous submucosal glands which produce mucus to help the food bolus move forward. It is made up of areolar connective tissue which links the mucosa to the muscularis;
- A muscularis has three layers of smooth muscle tissue: an outer longitudinal layer, a middle circular layer and an inner oblique layer;
- The external serosa lining the stomach is composed of simple squamous epithelium and areolar connective tissue, and forms part of the visceral peritoneum.

The mucosa is different in the fundus and body of the stomach and in the pyloric antrum.

- **The fundic mucosa**

These glands are composed of three types of cells:

- The main cells pepsinogen, which is the inactive form of pepsin, a proteolytic enzyme. The principal cells are found mainly in the basal regions of the gastric glands.
- The parietal cells (border cells), scattered throughout the main cells, secrete hydrochloric acid and intrinsic factor (which enables vitamin B12 to be absorbed in the small intestine).
- The few endocrine cells, the D cells, which secrete somatostatin.

- **The pyloric mucosa**

It has deep, narrow crypts and **two** types of cell.

- Collar mucus cells, found in the upper part, or "collar", of glands, produce a type of mucus. The precise function of this mucus is not yet known.
- Endocrine cells, G cells (secrete gastrin) and D cells (somatostatin) (Figure 2).

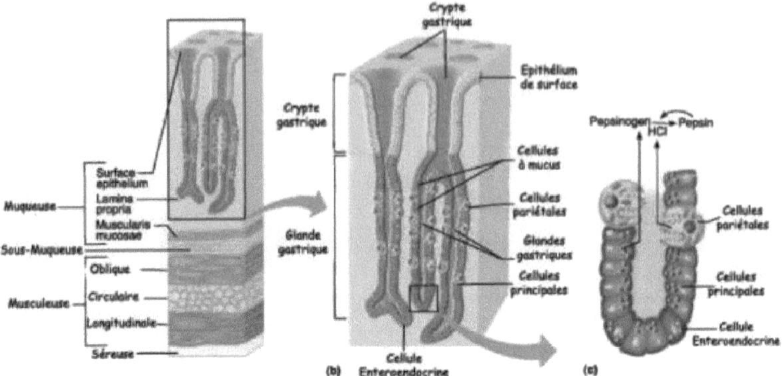

Figure 2: Histology of the stomach (Mennecier; 2022).

2.3. Physiology of the stomach

Before arriving in the stomach, food undergoes a number of transformations caused by chewing and saliva, and then passes into the resophagus. The bolus of food quickly finds its way back into the stomach and is called chyme.

The main role of the stomach is to transform food into a semi-liquid chyme so that it is acceptable to the intestine. The agent of this transformation is gastric juice, which is secreted by the gastric glands.

The stomach also secretes a mucus which forms a protective layer for the gastric mucosa against gastric acidity and which, by lubricating the ingesta, facilitates downstream passage.

2.3.1. Gastric juice

When food reaches the stomach, the stomach wall expands and the pH of the gastric contents increases because the proteins in the food have buffered some of the gastric acids. These changes trigger nerve impulses that stimulate the flow of gastric juice, a colourless, clear, acidic liquid (**pH between 1.5 and 2.5**) containing 7 g/l of dissolved substances, half organic and half mineral.

- **Mineral substances**
- Hydrochloric acid: secreted into the lumen of the glands by the parietal or border cells. It kills many bacteria ingested with food.
- Bicarbonates: secreted by mucus cells, helping to defend the gastric mucosa against acidity.
- **Organic substances**
- Mucus: secreted by mucus cells, forms a continuous film on the surface of the epithelium, providing physical and chemical protection acidity.
- Intrinsic factor: this is a glycoprotein secreted by parietal cells. It binds vitamin B12 (cobalamin) and transports it to the ileum, where it is absorbed.
- Pepsinogen I and II: secreted by the main cells, these are the inactive forms of pepsin which are activated by gastric acidity.
- Gastric lipase: secreted by the main cells. It is active in an acidic environment, and hydrolyses triglycerides into diglycerides and fatty acids.

2.3.2. Regulation of gastric acid secretion

Food intake stimulates acid secretion abruptly and steadily in a plateau for two hours, followed by a gradual return to basal levels; this process is also governed by nervous and hormonal mechanisms. HCl secretion is stimulated by three chemical substances, all of which act via second messenger systems (cAMP and Ca^{2+}).

— **Gastric secretion stimulants**

— Histamine: produced by histaminocytes or enterocromaffin-like cells (ECL), acts paracrine, binding to H2 receptors on parietal cells (adenylcyclase-coupled receptors) to increase intracellular cAMP.

— Gastrin: produced by G cells, acts endocrinally on the parietal cells themselves and on histaminocytes by stimulating the release of histamine. Gastrin receptors are coupled to a G protein which activates phospholipase C, leading to an increase in cytosolic Ca^{2+}.

— Acetylcholine: released by stimulation of the vagus nerve, it acts directly on parietal cells (M3 receptors) and indirectly by stimulating histaminocytes and gastrin cells.

Optimum acid secretion requires the synergistic action of all three mediators (Figure 3).

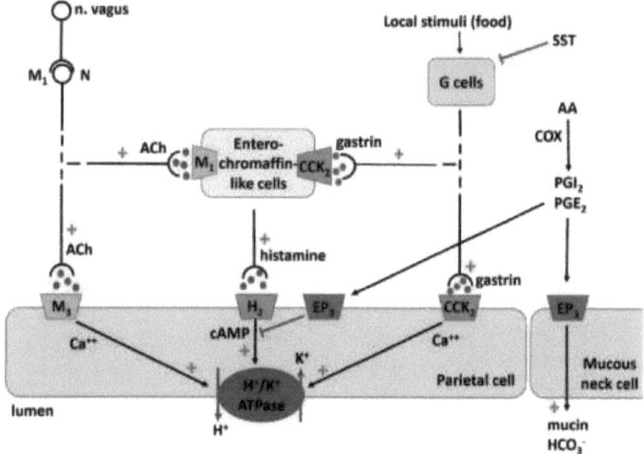

Figure 3: Gastric secretion (Artem Minalyan et al; 2017).

— **Gastric secretion inhibitors**

When chyme enters the duodenum, receptors in the duodenal wall react and trigger the enterogastric reflex, which inhibits gastric secretion. These include :

— Somatostatin: produced by D cells, acts paracrine and inhibits gastric secretion of all substances.

— Secretin: acts endocrinally, inhibiting gastric secretion and motility during the gastric phase of secretion.

— Prostaglandins: act by a paracrine route (receptors coupled to an adenylate cyclase-inhibiting G protein)

— Gastric inhibitor peptide (GIP): produced in the mucosa of the duodenum, inhibits the production of HCl (minor effect).

— Vasoactive intestinal peptide (VIP): produced in the mucosa of the duodenum, it inhibits the production of HCl in the stomach.

They all act directly on the parietal cell. There are three phases that play a role in gastric secretion, as follows:

— Cephalic phase: triggered by the thought, sight, smell, taste and contact of food in the mouth and resophagus. This stimulates the vagus nerve, releasing acetylcholine, which increases acid secretion from the stomach.

— Gastric phase: determines maximum acid secretion. It is triggered by the arrival of the food bolus in the stomach, where there is stimulation of the gastrin cells, which are the main mediator. H ions$^+$ also stimulate somatostatin secretion, which inhibits gastrin and histamine secretion, reducing acid output from the parietal cells.

— Intestinal phase: this completes the inhibition of acid secretion by gastric somatostatin. The arrival of acidic chyme in the duodenum leads to the secretion of secretin, somatostatin and GIP (gastric inhibitory peptide), which inhibit gastric acid secretion by endocrine action.

2.4. Gastric pathologies

2.4.1. Gastroesophageal reflux disease

Gastro-resophageal reflux disease (GERD) is a physiological reflex inducing acid reflux from the stomach into the resophagus. GERD becomes pathological when these acid refluxes become too frequent and significant, and can cause lesions, leading to peptic resophagitis (Figure 4).

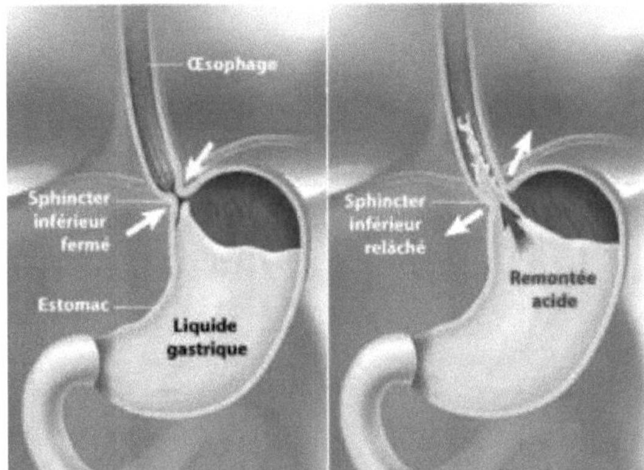

Figure 4. pathological mechanism of GERD (Mohamed A El-Mahdy; 2017).

The typical signs of GERD are retrosternal burning and acid regurgitation, which may be associated with atypical (less specific) signs such as chest pain, cough, asthma or dental erosions.

GERD is favoured by lying down or bending over, and mainly by being overweight. Other contributing factors are alcohol, smoking, pregnancy, the presence of a hiatal hernia and certain drugs via different mechanisms (ascorbic acid, alendronate, potassium chloride, tetracycline, etc.).

Diagnosis is clinical in most cases, but additional tests are required in certain situations (over 50 years of age, relapse or resistance to antisecretory treatment, warning signs such as weight loss or deterioration in general condition and dysphagia, and in cases of atypical symptoms). A resogastroduodenal fibroscopy (FOGD) or resophageal pH-metry is then performed.

The first-line treatment is non-medical and is based on hygiene and dietary rules, limiting overeating and late meals, and weight loss if necessary.

2.4.2. Hiatus hernia

Hiatal hernia is defined as the intermittent or permanent passage of part of the stomach through the resophageal orifice of the diaphragm or resophageal hiatus.

There are two types of hiatus hernia:

- Hiatal hernia caused by the cardia sliding into the thorax (85% of cases)
- Rolling or para-resophageal hiatal hernia (10% of cases), when the stomach slides along the resophagus above the diaphragm, without altering the position of the cardia (Figure 5).

Mixed (rolling and sliding) hiatal hernias occur in 5% of cases (Figure 5,6).

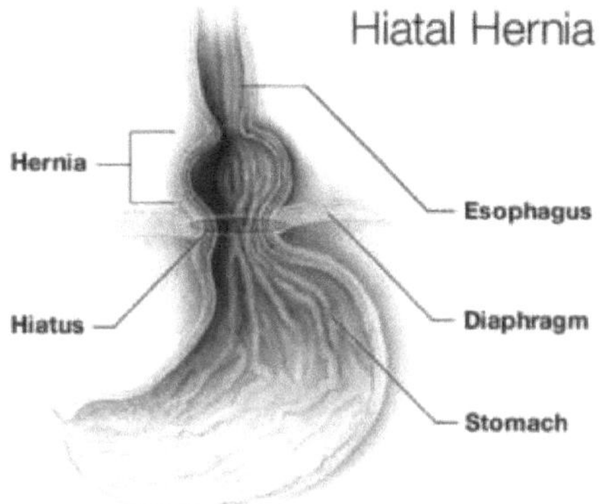

Figure 5. hiatal hernia (Rishi K et al; 2015).

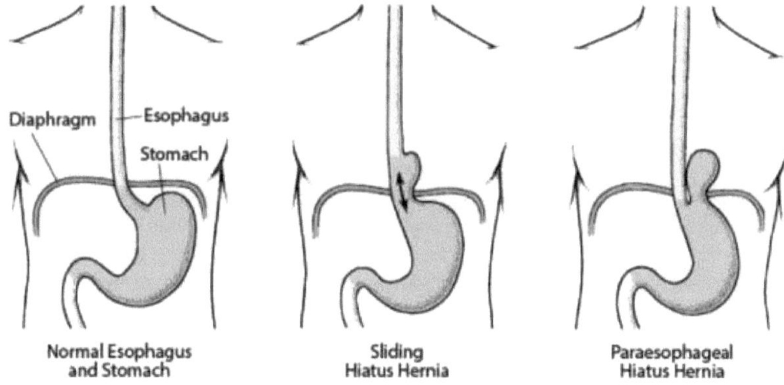

Figure 6. Types of hiatal hernia (Rishi K et al; 2015.

This is the most common lesion of the digestive tract, affecting 20 to 60% of the population in France, with a good prognosis and rarely complicated. It is triggered when the means of fixation of the resophagus and stomach fail. It can be asymptomatic or cause signs of GERD, dyspepsia or dysphagia. Treatment is primarily medical, followed by surgery if this fails, taking into account the risk/benefit balance.

2.4.3. Peptic ulcer

Ulcers can occur in the gastric or duodenal mucosa, in areas of inflammation known as gastritis, duodenitis or bulbitis. They are diagnosed endoscopically on the basis of signs of redness, redness and swelling of the mucosa, combined with histological diagnosis by biopsy (Figure 7).

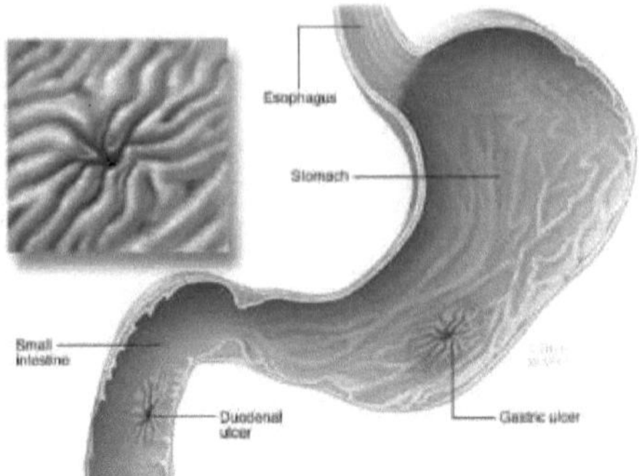

Figure 7. Peptic ulcer disease (Mayo clinic; 2022).

The ulcer itself corresponds to a worsening of these areas of inflammation, with a loss of mucosal substance least 0.5 cm in diameter reaching the muscularis mucosae. These lesions occur in two-thirds of cases in the stomach, but can also occur throughout the digestive tract.

Clinical symptoms typically include recurrent episodes of pain in the epigastric cavity, which may also be associated with nausea, vomiting and retrosternal burning. When the ulcer is complicated by perforation or haemorrhage, it is associated with acute abdominal pain, haematemesis or melena, anaemia and even hypovolaemic shock.

The worldwide prevalence of gastritis is closely linked to that of Helicobacter pylori (HP). Its colonisation is almost systematically accompanied by chronic gastritis, which only regresses 6 to 24 months after eradication of the bacteria, and is present in the vast majority of cases when an ulcer discovered (85 to 95%). However, most of these patients will not develop an ulcer, and carriage of the bacterium will remain asymptomatic: 5 to 15% of H. pylori-infected subjects will develop an ulcer, i.e. 3 to 8 times more than in H. pylori-negative patients.

H. pylori and NSAIDs alone are responsible for 85-90% of ulcers.

2.4.4. Gsophagus of Barrett or endobrachyssophagus

Endobrachyresophagus (EBO), also known as Barrett's resophagus, is a metaplasia of the resophageal mucosa. Normally, the mucosa is of the epidermolysis type and covers the entire resophagus. It is then replaced distally by an intestinal-type glandular mucosa following a repair process. This process is induced by the inflammatory lesions caused by GERD (Figure 8).

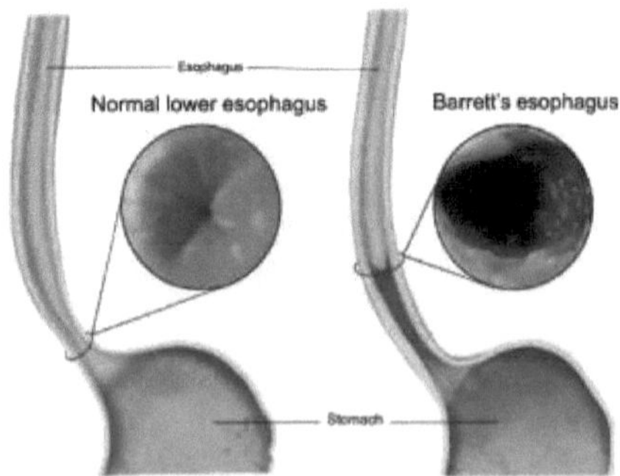

Figure 8. Gsophagus of BARRETT (Spechler SJ et al; 2014).

This transformation is not trivial, and can progress to high-grade dysplasia and then adenocarcinoma, with an estimated probability of between 0.2 and 2% in patients with OBE. OBE is classically associated with hiatal hernia, and is present in 5-15% of patients with symptomatic GERD, indicating the need for endoscopic examination. It can also develop in patients with no signs of reflux. It is only diagnosed by endoscopy, which is not routinely performed, which is why the prevalence of OBE is not precisely known.
The risk factors identified are chronic and long-standing reflux, smoking, age, android obesity, and gender (predominantly middle-aged men).

2.4.5. ZOLLINGER-ELLISON syndrome

Zollinger-Ellison syndrome (ZES) develops following the appearance of a gastrinoma. This is an endocrine tumour that causes an increase in gastrin secretion, resulting in gastric acid hypersecretion. Gastrinomas are generally found in the duodenum, pancreas or abdominal lymph nodes, and are diagnosed by imaging.
This very rare phenomenon leads to severe peptic disease in the form of multiple severe ulcers or resophagitis. The incidence is low: 1-2/1,000,000 in the general population.
SZE is diagnosed when fasting gastrinemia is greater than 10 times normal, associated with a gastric pH of less than 2. Treatment is symptomatic with PPIs and curative as soon as possible with surgical removal of the gastrinoma.

3. Classification

Digestive tract medicines are classified according to the mechanisms of action listed below:

> Neutralisation of gastric acid (antacids)

- Systemic (absorbable) : $NaHCO_3$ and sodium citrate.
- Non-systemic (non-absorbable): $Mg(OH)_2$, $CaCO_3$, aluminium hydroxide gel.

> Reduction in gastric acid secretion (antisecretory)

- Proton pump : Omeprazole, Lansoprazole and Pantoprazole.
- Prostaglandin analogues: Misoprostol.
- H2 antihistamines: Cimetidine, Ranitidine and Famotidine.
- Anticholinergics: Pirenzepine, Propantheline and Oxyphenonium.

> **Ulcer protectors (gastric topicals)** : Sucralfate, colloidal Bismuth subcitrate (CBS).

4. Antacids

Antacids have been used for centuries in the treatment of patients suffering from dyspepsia and acid-related disorders. They formed the basis of treatment for acid-related disorders until the advent of H2-receptor antagonists and proton pump inhibitors.

Antacids act directly in the gastric lumen by neutralising the hydrochloric acid secreted by the parietal cells. They are defined as contact antacids, and enable the gastric PH to be modulated by increasing it.

The usual forms found combine aluminium hydroxide and magnesium hydroxide. Other formulations include bicarbonates, phosphates or silicates. The difference in composition gives antacids varying neutralising capacities (Table I).

Table I. Main antacids.

Molecule INN	Trade name and pharmaceutical form	Chemical structure and scientific name
Bicarbonate de sodium	***Alka-Seltzer®*** (325 mg par comprimé)	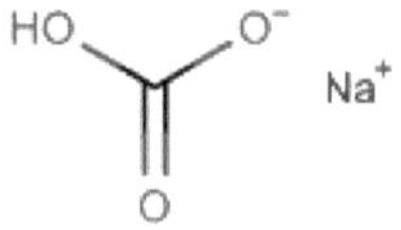 HO–C(=O)–O^- Na^+
Carbonate de calcium	***TUMS®*** (500 mg par comprimé)	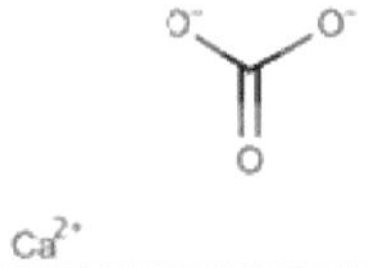 O^-–C(=O)–O^- Ca^{2+}

Table I. Main antacids (continued).

Molecule INN	Trade name and pharmaceutical form	Chemical structure and scientific name
Carbonate de magnésium	***Phillips' Milk of Magnesia®*** (400 mg par comprimé)	Mg^{2+} CO_3^{2-}
Hydroxyde de magnésium	***AZYM®*** (400 mg par comprimé)	HO–Mg–OH
Hydroxyde d'aluminium	***GASTRALUGEL®*** (500 mg par comprimé)	Al^{3+} OH^- OH^- OH^-
Phosphate d'aluminium	***PHOSPHALUGEL®*** Suspension buvable	Al^{3+} PO_4^{3-}

Antacids have developed from the hydroxides and carbonates of Group II and III metals, and the bicarbonates of alkali metals. All antacids contain at least one of the following metals: aluminium, calcium, magnesium, sodium, potassium or bismuth.

4.1. Absorbable antacids

They are soluble, easily absorbed and capable of producing systemic electrolyte abnormalities. Their properties are as follows:

— Absorbed into the systemic circulation ;

— They have a cationic group which does not form insoluble basic compounds with a bicarbonate ion (HCO_3), so that HCO_3^- can be absorbed;

— Rebound phenomenon: This is a physiological response to the alkalinisation of the environment, which activates the secretion of hydrochloric acid (HCl). It is triggered by stimulation of gastrin production and the direct effect of calcium on the parietal cells of the stomach mucosa. Many drugs in this group contribute to the mechanical distension of the stomach wall, which in itself is a powerful acid stimulant;

— Short-lasting effects: short-lasting effects increase dosing intervals, which increases the risk of complications;

— Alters the acid-base balance in favour of metabolic alkalosis;

— Reduced gastric and intestinal emptying (constipation) ;

— Adverse effects on pregnant women and the elderly.

4.2. Non-absorbable antacids

They help avoid the complications mentioned above. Properties include:

- Compounds that are not absorbed into the systemic circulation.
- Their anionic group neutralises the hydrogen ions (H^+) in gastric acid. This releases their cationic group, which combines with HCO_3^- from the pancreas to form an insoluble basic

compound that is excreted in the faeces;

- These agents do not produce metabolic alkalosis;
- Accumulation of calcium (Ca^{2+}), magnesium (Mg^{2+}) and aluminium (Al^{2+}). Dangerous in cases of renal insufficiency, as aluminium compounds are contraindicated in cases of renal insufficiency.
- Encephalopathy and arthropathy Occurs during chronic administration of compounds mainly based on bismuth (Bi^{3+}).
- Nephrolithiasis: occurs with compounds containing silicon.

4.3. Lead study: Sodium bicarbonate NaHCO3

4.3.1. Chemical synthesis

Sodium bicarbonate is synthesised using the Solvay process. The Solvay process involves the reaction of sodium chloride, ammonia and carbon dioxide in water.

$$NaCl + H2O + CO2 + NH3 \quad NH4Cl + NaHCO3$$

The carbon dioxide required for the reaction is produced by heating ("calcining") the limestone to 950-1100°C, and the calcium oxide produced is used to recover ammonia from the ammonium chloride.

4.3.2. Quality control

1. Physico-chemical properties

Sodium bicarbonate is a white or almost white, slightly granular, hygroscopic powder. It is easily soluble in water and practically insoluble in 96% ethanol.

2. Identification

Dissolve 1 g of sodium carbonate in water R and make up to 10 ml with the same solvent. The solution is strongly alkaline

— The solution prepared in the identification gives the carbonate reaction.

— The solution prepared in the identification gives the sodium reaction.

3. Test

- Test for loss on drying of chlorides and sulphates.

4. Dosage

Potentiometric titration with hydrochloric acid.

4.5. Mechanism of action

Antacids are weak bases that react with gastric hydrochloric acid to form a salt and water.

However, the acid-neutralising capacity of different antacid formulations varies widely, depending on the speed at which they are dissolved (tablet or liquid), their solubility in water, the speed at which they react with acid and the speed at which they are emptied from the stomach.

> Sodium bicarbonate (sodium bicarbonate, *ALKA SELTZER®*) reacts rapidly with hydrochloric acid (HCl) to produce carbon dioxide and sodium chloride. The formation of carbon causes gastric distension and gas emissions. Unreacted alkali is readily absorbed and may cause metabolic alkalosis when administered in high doses or to patients with renal failure.

> Calcium carbonate is less soluble and reacts more slowly than sodium bicarbonate with HCl to form carbon dioxide and calcium chloride (CaCl2). Like sodium bicarbonate, calcium carbonate can cause colic or metabolic alkalosis.

> Preparations containing magnesium hydroxide or aluminium react slowly with HCl to form magnesium chloride or aluminium and water. As no gas is produced, there is no eructation. Metabolic alkalosis is also rare due to the efficiency of the neutralisation reaction.

> As unabsorbed magnesium can cause osmotic diarrhoea and aluminium constipation, these agents are commonly administered together in patented formulations (e.g. *GELUSIL®* , *MAALOX®* , *MYLANTA®*) to minimise the impact on intestinal function.

4.6. Indications

- Symptoms of heartburn in GERD ;
- Duodenal and gastric ulcers ;
- Stress gastritis ;
- Pancreatic insufficiency ;
- Non-ulcer dyspepsia ;
- Diarrhoea caused by acids bile acids ;
- Biliary reflux ;
- Constipation ;
- Osteoporosis ;
- Urinary alkalinisation ;
- Phosphate binding in chronic renal renal failure.

4.7. Undesirable effects

Adverse effects are greatest in infants and the elderly. Chronic use of antacids in this population is not recommended for safety reasons.

- **Aluminium hydroxide**

The use of aluminium is associated with an increased risk of toxicity in people from renal failure and in infants. This is manifested by :

- Osteopenia ;
- Microcytic anaemia ;
- Neurotoxicity ;
- Osteomalacia ;
- Constipation ;
- Fecal impaction ;
- Nausea ;
- Vomiting ;
- Abdominal cramps ;
- Hypomagnesaemia ;
- Hypophosphatemia.

> Calcium carbonate

The adverse reactions often observed with this group antacids are as follows:

- Abdominal pain ;
- Anorexia ;
- Constipation ;
- Acid rebound ;
- Nausea ;
- Vomiting ;
- Flatulence ;
- Xerostomia ;
- Headaches ;
- Hypercalcaemia ;
- Hypophosphatemia.

5. Proton pump inhibitors

Proton pump inhibitors (PPIs) are a therapeutic class that has revolutionised the treatment of gastric acid-related disorders in the digestive tract.

PPIs belong to a group of molecules whose action targets the proton pump in gastric parietal cells.

5.5. History of discovery

In 1973, a series of studies directed by *G. Sachs* demonstrated the presence of a membrane transporter capable of transporting an H ion$^+$ using a K ion$^+$ as a counterion, and whose operation is essentially based on a phosphorylation mechanism. The results of these studies led to the naming of this transporter the H^+ /K^+ ATPase pump, more commonly known as the proton pump, which accounts for more than 85% of membrane proteins in parietal cells and is located exclusively in the gastric tract. At the end of the 1970s, research into the antiviral potential of PYRIDYLTHIOACETAMIDE revealed the anti-secretory nature of this compound. TIMOPRAZOLE, a benzimidazole pyridylmethylsulphoxide with a similar structure, was tested on the H /$K^{+ +}$ ATPase pump, confirming the anti-secretory properties of sulphoxides.

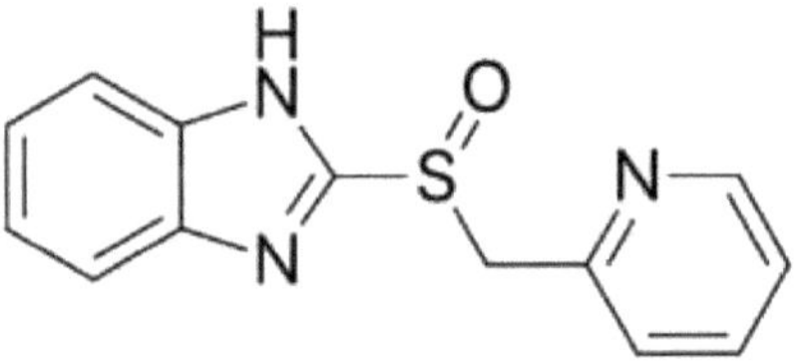

Figure 9: structure of Timoprazole.

Research then focused on optimisation studies by substitution and addition of adicals to the benzimidazole and pyridine rings in order obtain ionisation constants adjusted to a pH below 4 that were specific to the gastric environment. Thusin 1989, OMEPRAZOLE became the first specific proton pump inhibitor on the market and the leader of a new therapeutic class. This was followed in chronological order by LANSOPRAZOLE in 1990, PANTOPRAZOLE in 1995, RABEPRAZOLE in 1998 and finally ESOMEPRAZOLE in 2000 (table II).

Table II. Main proton pump inhibitors.

Molecule INN	Trade name and pharmaceutical form	Chemical structure and scientific name
Oméprazole	***PRILOSEC ® MOPRAL®*** Gélule à 10 et 20 mg	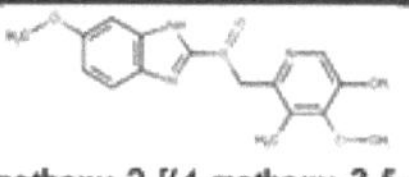 methoxy-2-[(4-methoxy-3,5-dimethylpyridin-2-yl)methyl sulfinyl]-1H-benzimidazole
Lansoprazole	***PREVACID®*** Comprimé à 15 mg	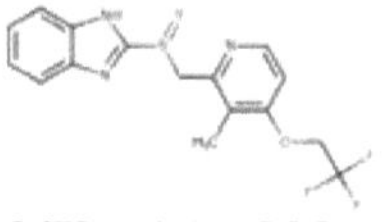 2-[[[3-methyl-4-(2,2,2-tri fluoroethoxy)-2-pyridinyl] methyl]sulfinyl]-1H-benz imidazole
Pantoprazole	***PROTONIX®*** Comprimé à 40 mg	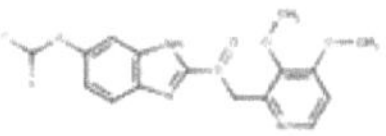 5-(difluoromethoxy)-2-[(3,4-dimethoxypyridin-2-yl)me thylsulfinyl]-1H-benzimi dazole
Rabéprazole	***PARIET®*** Comprimé à 20 mg	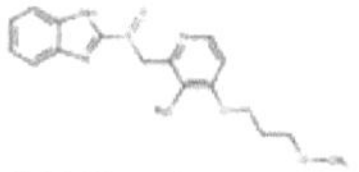 2-({[4-(3-methoxypropoxy)-3-methylpyridin-2-yl]methy l}sulfinyl)-1H-benzimidazole
Ésoméprazole	***NEXIUM®*** Comprimé à 20mg et 40 mg	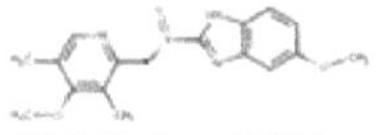 (S)-5-Methoxy-2-[[(4-me thoxy-3,5-dimethyl-2-py ridinyl)methyl]sulfinyl]-1H-benzimidazole

5.6. Lead study

Omeprazole: *MOPRAL®*

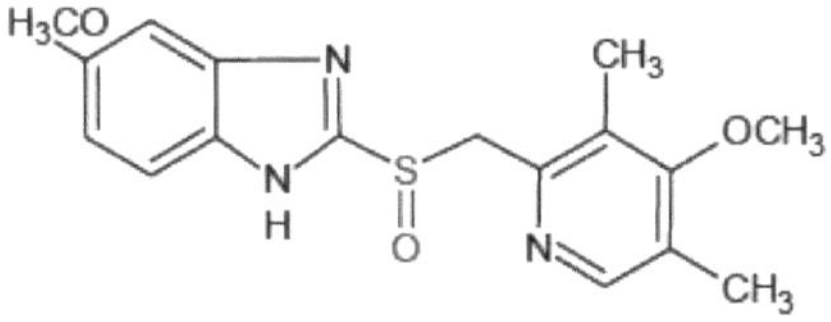

H_3CO N H S O N CH_3 OCH_3 CH_3

Figure 10. Structure of Omeprazole.

Originally approved by the FDA in 1989, Omeprazole is a proton pump inhibitor used to treat disorders associated with gastric acidity. These disorders may include gastro- resophageal reflux disease (GERD), peptic ulcer disease and other conditions characterised by excessive gastric acid secretion.

It was the first clinically useful drug in its class, and its approval was followed by the formulation of many other proton pump inhibitor drugs . Omeprazole is generally effective and well tolerated, making it popular for use in both children and adults.

5.6.1. Chemical synthesis

Omeprazole is synthesised by a cyclisation reaction between 4- methoxybenzene -1,2-diamine and potassium O-ethylcarbonodithioate in the presence of carbon disulphide and potassium ethanoate to form 5-methoxy-1H-1,3-benzimidazole -2-thiolate, the latter undergoes a nucleophilic substitution reaction with 1-(chloromethyl)-3-methoxy-2,4-dimethylbenzene with the release of potassium chloride to produce 5-methoxy-2-{[(3-methoxy-2,4- dimethylphenyl) methyl]sulphanyl}-1H-1,3-benzimidazole, which is oxidised by m-chloroperbenzoic acid to Omeprazole.

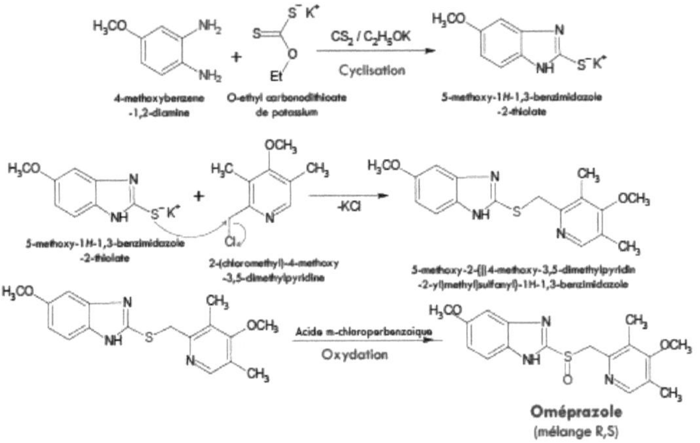

Figure 11. Chemical synthesis of Omeprazole.

1. Physico-chemical properties

Omeprazole is a white or almost white hygroscopic powder. It is very slightly soluble in water, fairly soluble in methanol and practically insoluble in heptane.

2. Identification

- Optical angle of rotation: - 0.1 0°to + 0.1 0°.
- Infrared absorption spectrophotometry
- Atomic absorption spectrometry

3. Test

- Assay of related substances by liquid chromatography.
- Test for loss on drying, heavy metals and sulphuric ash.

4. Dosage

Liquid chromatography.

5.7. Business structure relationship

The currently available gastric proton pump inhibitors all retain the same key chemical features present in Omeprazole, indicating that the structural requirements for achieving irreversible inhibition of the gastric ATPase enzyme are precisely defined.

Omeprazole's three main structural features (i.e. the substituted pyridine ring, the substituted benzimidazole and the methylsulfinyl linking group, by which these two ring systems are attached to each other) are essential either to generate the active form from its inactive prodrug precursor or to bind irreversibly to the H+/K+ ATPase enzyme.

Although many compounds lack substituents on the benzimidazole ring, the presence of electron-donating groups in the 5-position, such as methoxy (omeprazole) and difluoromethoxy (pantoprazole), has also helped achieve an optimal balance between chemical stability and reactivity. On the other hand, the presence of electron-withdrawing substituents in this position, such as nitro, methylsulphinyl and trifluoromethyl, increases the basicity of the benzimidmole ring to the extent that the behaviour of these compounds is dominated by activation at neutral pH, resulting in compounds with low chemical stability and limited practical value.

On the other hand, increasing the nucleophilic nature of the pyridine ring, by incorporating electron-donating substituents, improves rate of attack on the C-2 position of the benzimidazole group and thus promotes acid-catalysed rearrangement to the active species. This electronic characteristic is present in omeprazole (3,5-dimethyl-4-methoxy) and pantoprazole (2,3- dimethoxy), it is associated with an increased lipophilic character in compounds substituted by benzimidazole 4-fluoroalkyl, such as lansoprazole (2,2,2-trifluoroethyloxy).

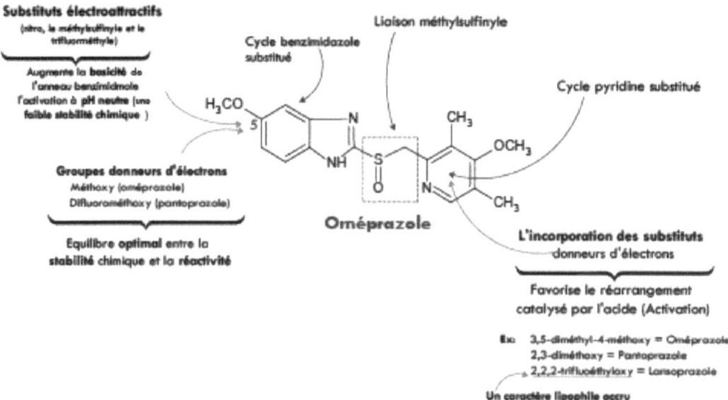

Figure 12. Structure-activity relationship of Omeprazole.

The 3-methoxypropoxy substituent on the pyridyl group of rabeprazole is a particularly strong electron donor, but the resulting increase in reactivity in this case is mitigated by formulation as a sodium salt increase chemical stability.

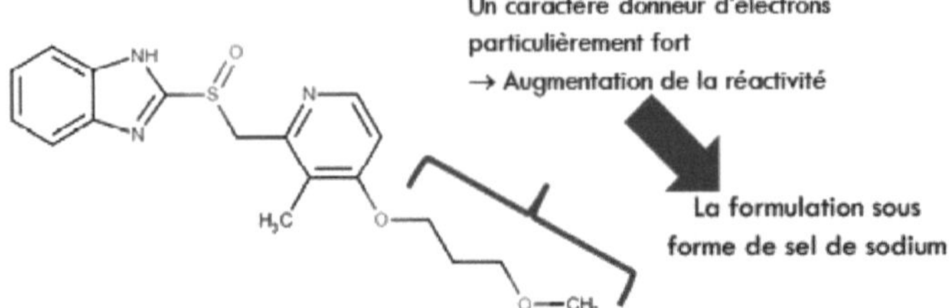

Figure 13. Structure of Rabeprazole.

5.8. Mechanism of action

A better understanding of the mechanism of action of proton pump inhibitors requires a more in-depth understanding of the structure of the target.

The proton pump is located in the membrane of the secretory canaliculi of the parietal cell. Its structure comprises two subunits, α and β. The a subunit represents the active structure, fulfilling both enzymatic and transmembrane ion transport functions. The β subunit plays a structural role, maintaining the structure and folding the a subunit.

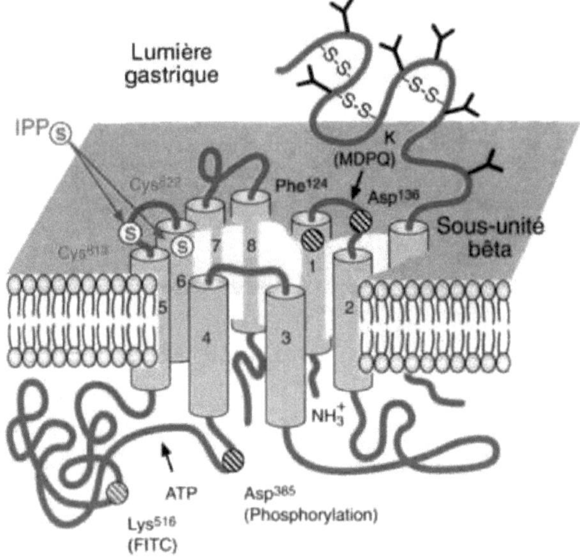

Figure 14. Proton pump.

Proton pump inhibitors all act by inhibiting gastric acid secretion by blocking the enzymatic activity of adenosine triphosphates, which provides the energy required for the transmembrane passage of ions.

Their mechanism of action is divided into three main stages:

> Accumulation

Proton pump inhibitors are prodrugs. When administered orally, proton pump inhibitors are absorbed from the intestine and enter the bloodstream. They diffuse by blood transport and are found in inactive form in the cytoplasm of the parietal cell.

The chemical structure and electrically neutral state give these prodrugs a very lipophilic, weak base status, which facilitates their passage across the ductal membrane. The proton pump inhibitors then accumulate in inactive form in the acidic canalicular space.

> Activation

Thanks to the acidic pH of the canalicular space, the sulphoxide group is reduced to sulphenamide, which is the active form of the drug responsible for its inhibitory action. The sulphenamide ring has a reactive sulphur which forms an irreversible covalent bond with the thiol group of the free amino terminal cysteines of the a subunit.

This protonation step plays a key role in the specific mechanism of action of proton pump inhibitors. Protonation is only possible in the canaliculus of the parietal cell, as this is the only biological compartment where the pH is low enough to both accumulation and activation of the inactive form of the drug.

> Inhibition

Inhibition of the proton pump is the result of an irreversible covalent bond formed at the luminal surface of the parietal cell, between the sulphenamide function of a PPI and the thiol group of cysteine 813 of subunit a, the H+ ion transport zone.

The resulting inhibition is total and lasts around 24 hours. This depends in fact on the time required for the physiological synthesis a new proton pump, which is of the order of 18 to 24 hours.

5.9. Indications

— Curative and preventive treatment of active gastric or duodenal ulcers, in combination with antibiotic therapy as part of Helicobacter pylori eradication.

— Curative and preventive treatment of erosive resophagitis following gastroresophageal reflux.

— Symptomatic treatment of gastro-resophageal reflux disease.

— Curative and preventive treatment of gastric or duodenal ulcers induced by non-steroidal anti-inflammatory drugs, particularly in patients at risk.

— Treatment of Zollinger-Ellison syndrome.

5.10. Undesirable effects

Generally speaking, these drugs do not have any major or recurring adverse effects, but they do cause some symptoms which are generally transient, particularly when treatment is initiated, and reversible when treatment is stopped.

The most common side effects are gastrointestinal, with cases of nausea or vomiting, flatulence, constipation, abdominal pain and diarrhoea.

6. Prostaglandin analogues

Prostaglandins have antisecretory effects on gastric acid. As well as inhibiting the activity of adenylyl cyclase in parietal cells, which leads to a reduction in gastric acid secretion, prostaglandins stimulate the secretion of mucus and bicarbonate in adjacent superficial cells.

However, PGE1 suffers from a number drawbacks that have prevented its use as a therapeutic treatment for peptic ulcer disease. The main problems are the lack oral activity, short duration of action and a variety of adverse effects.
The only oral prostaglandin available in the United States is Misoprostol. The oral carboxylic acid ester is hydrolysed to a pharmacologically active carboxylic acid. It is a synthetic analogue of prostaglandin E1, in which structural modifications are made to prevent rapid metabolic conversion to inactive products (Table III).

Table III. Main prostaglandin analogues.

Molecule DCI	Trade name and form pharmaceutical	Chemical structure and scientific name
Misoprostol	**CYTOTEC ®** Comprimé à100 ug et 200 ug	(11α,13E)-(+)-11α,16-Dihydroxy -16-methyl-9-oxo-prost-13-en-1-oic acid methyl ester

6.1. Lead study

Misoprostol: *CYTOTEC* ®

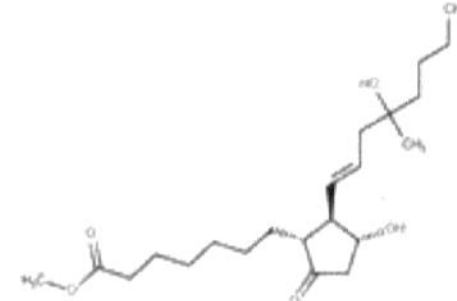

Figure 14. Structure of Misoprostol.

Misoprostol is a prostaglandin analogue used to reduce the risk NSAID-related ulcers.
Stimulation of prostaglandin receptors in the stomach reduces gastric acid secretion, while stimulation of these receptors in the uterus and cervix can increase the strength and frequency of contractions and reduce cervical tone.

6.1.1 Chemical synthesis

Misoprostol can be synthesised by a reaction called cuprate coupling, using an organocuprate reagent and a cyclopenteneheptanoate derivative.

methyl 7-(3-hydroxy-5-oxocyclopent-1-en-1-yl)heptanoate + Réactif organocuprate lithié → (Couplage Cuprate) → Misoprostol

Figure 15. Chemical synthesis of Misoprostol.

6.1.2. Quality control

1. Physico-chemical properties

Misoprostol is an oily, clear, colourless or yellowish, hygroscopic liquid. It is practically insoluble in water, soluble in 96% ethanol and fairly soluble in acetonitrile.

2. **Identification**

Infrared absorption spectrophotometry

3. **Test**

- Assay of related substances by liquid chromatography.
- Test for loss on drying, heavy metals and sulphuric ash.

4. **Dosage**

Liquid chromatography.

6.2. Mechanism of action

Stimulation of prostaglandin receptors in the stomach reduces gastric acid secretion, while stimulation of these receptors in the uterus and cervix can increase the strength and frequency of contractions and reduce cervical tone.

Activation of the EP3 receptor has been proposed as the receptor responsible for antisecretory and cytoprotective effects as well as uterine contractions, while the EP receptor has been postulated as the receptor responsible for diarrhoea. Misoprostol acts as a prodrug whose a-methyl ester must be hydrolysed to the free acid by esterase activity. The prodrug is selective for the EP3 receptor (figure 16).

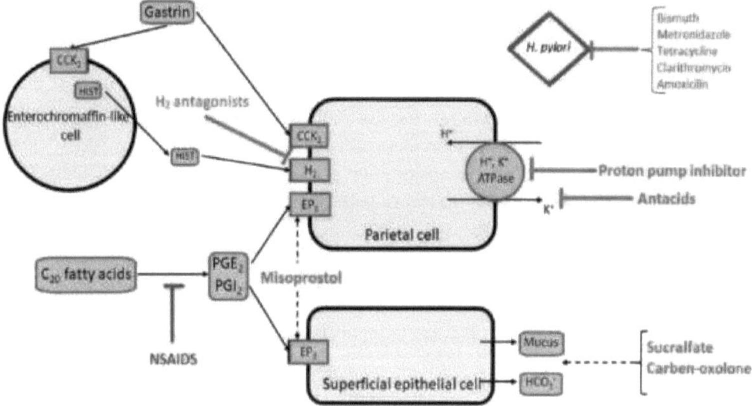

Figure 16. Mechanism of action of Misoprostol.

6.3. Indications

Misoprostol is indicated in tablet form to reduce the risk NSAID-induced gastric ulcers, but not duodenal ulcers in high-risk patients.

Misoprostol is also formulated in combination with Diclofenac to treat the symptoms of osteoarthritis or rheumatoid arthritis in patients at high risk gastric ulcers. Misoprostol is used off-label for the management of miscarriage and the prevention of postpartum haemorrhage.

6.4. Undesirable effects

The most common side effects are abdominal pain, nausea, flatulence, headache, dyspepsia, vomiting and constipation.

7. H2 antihistamines

Selective histamine type 2 receptor antagonists/blockers (H2 blockers) are widely used in the treatment of acid-related diseases, including duodenal and gastric ulcers, gastro-resophageal reflux disease and common heartburn.

Histamine or 4(5-)(2-aminoethyl) imidazole is a biogenic amine synthesised from L-histidine exclusively by L-histidine decarboxylase.

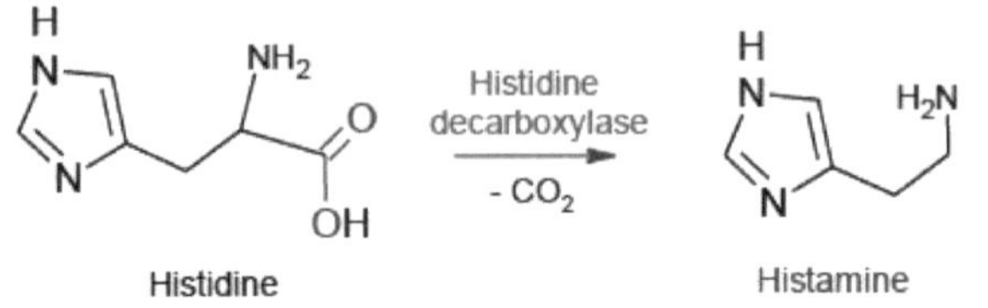

Figure 17. Histamine biosynthesis.

The effect of histamine is regulated by four types of receptor: H1, H2, H3 and H4. Histamine receptors are G protein-coupled receptors, which are proteins with 7 transmembrane chambers.

The four histamine receptor subtypes differ in their expression, localisation, primary structure, precise signal transduction processes and physiological function.

The H2 receptor is a receptor coupled to the Gs protein; when the receptor is stimulated by the activation an adenylate cyclase, the intracellular concentration cyclic AMP increases. Cyclic AMP activates the hydrogen-potassium pump, causing the secretion of hydrogen ions.

Drugs pharmacological action mainly involves antagonising the action of histamine at its H2 receptors are used therapeutically in the treatment of acid-peptic disorders, including heartburn, gastro-resophageal reflux disease, erosive resophagitis, gastric and duodenal ulcers and gastric acid hypersecretory pathological diseases such as Zollinger-Ellison syndrome (table IV).

Table IV: Main H2 antihistamine molecules.

Molecule DCI	Trade name and form pharmaceutical	Chemical structure and scientific name
Cimétidine	***TAGAMET®*** **Comprimé à 200 et 400 mg**	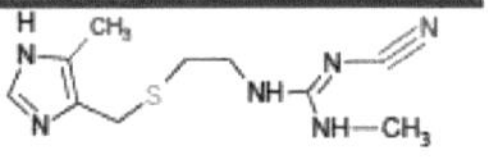 **1-Cyano-3-méthyl-2-(2-{[(4-méthyl-1H-imidazol-5-yl)méthyl]sulfanyl}éthyl) guanidine**
Famotidine	***PEPCID®*** **Comprimé à 20 et 40 mg** **Solution injectable á 10mg/1mL** **Non enregistré en Algérie**	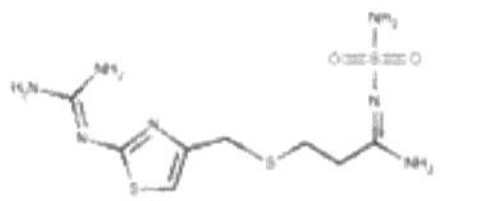 **3-[({2-[(diaminomethylidene)amino]-1,3-thiazol-4-yl}methyl)sulfanyl]-N'-sulfamoylpropanimidamide**

Table IV: Main H2 antihistamine molecules (continued).

Molecule DCI	Trade name and form pharmaceutical	Chemical structure and scientific name
Nizatidine	***AXID®*** Gélule á 150 mg **Arrêt de commercialisation**	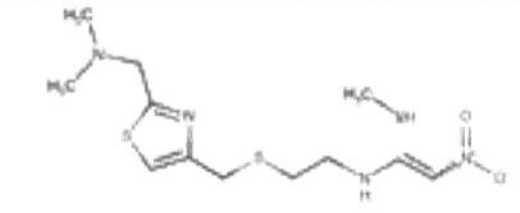 N-{2-[({2-[(Diméthylamino)méthyl]-1,3-thiazol-4-yl}méthyl) sulfanyl]éthyl}-N'-méthyl-2-nitro-1,1-éthènediamine
Ranitidine	***ZANTAC®*** Gélule á 150 et 300 mg Solution injectable á 50mg/2mL **Arrêt de commercialisation**	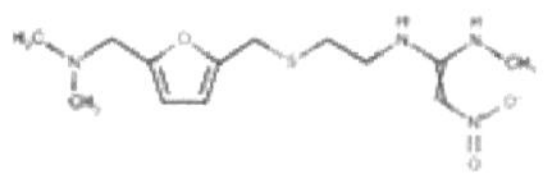 N-{2-[({5-[(Diméthylamino)méthyl]-2-furyl}méthyl) sulfanyl]éthyl}-N'-méthyl-2-nitro-1,1-éthènediamine
Roxatidine	***ROXANE®*** Gélule á 75mg Non enregistré en Algérie	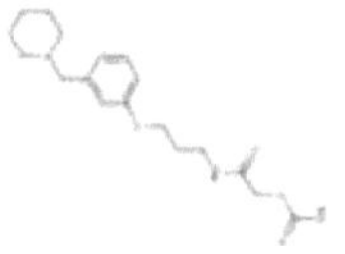 [(3-{3-[(piperidin-1-yl)methyl]phenoxy} propyl)carbamoyl] methyl acetate

7.1. Lead study

TAGAMET® **cimetidine**

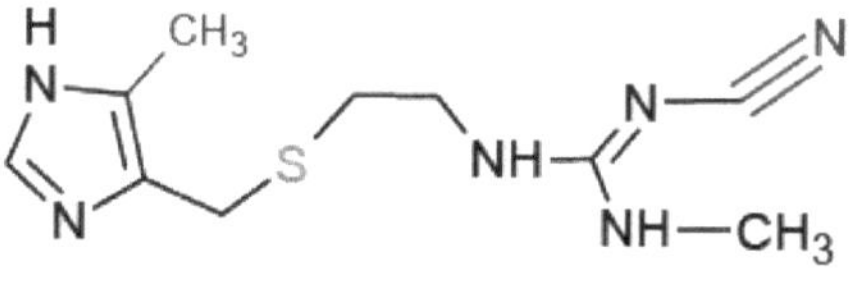

Figure 18. Chemical structure of cimetidine.

7.1.1. Chemical synthesis

It can be summarised as follows:

1- The reaction of 2-chloroacetoacetic ether with two moles of formamide gives 4-carbethoxy-5-methylimidazol.

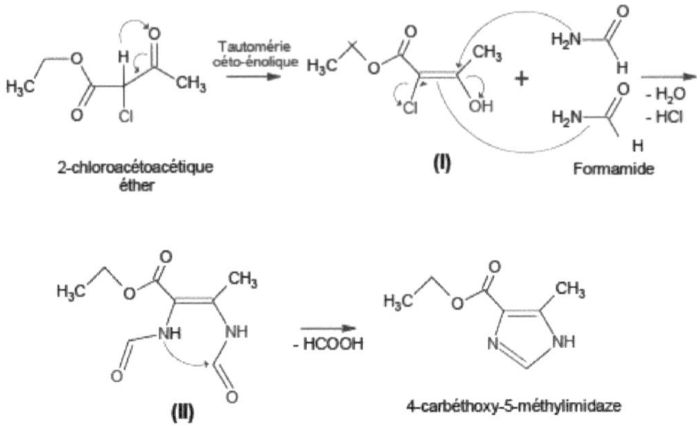

Tautomérie
céto-énolique
- H2O
- HCl
2-chloroacétoacétique éther
(I)
Formamide
- HCOOH
(II)
4-carbéthoxy-5-méthylimidaze

Figure 19. Chemical synthesis of cimetidine.

2- Reduction of this product with sodium in liquid ammonia gives 4-hydroxymethyl-5-methylimidazol.

Na/NH3
Reduction
- CH3CH2OH
4-carbéthoxy-5-méthylimidaze
4-hydroxyméthyle-5-méthylimidazol

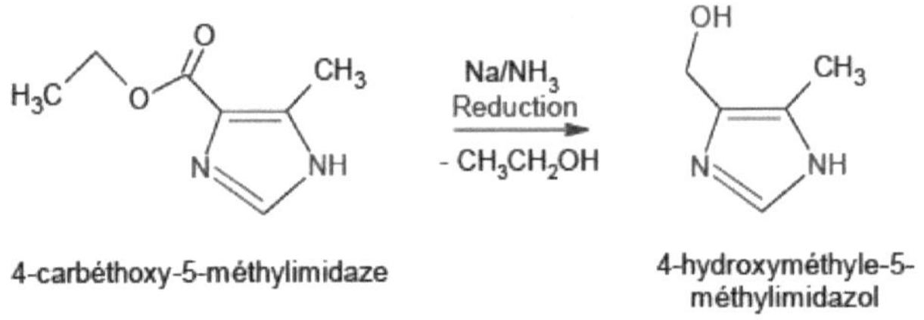

Figure 20: Chemical synthesis of cimetidine (continued).

The alcohol hydrochloride obtained is reacted with 2-mercaptoethylamine hydrochloride to produce 4-(2-aminomethyl)- thiomethyl5-methylimidazol dihydrochloride.

3-

- H2O
4-hydroxyméthyle-5-méthylimidazol
2-mercaptoéthylamine
4-(2-aminométhyl)-thiométhyl5-méthylimidazol dihydrochloride

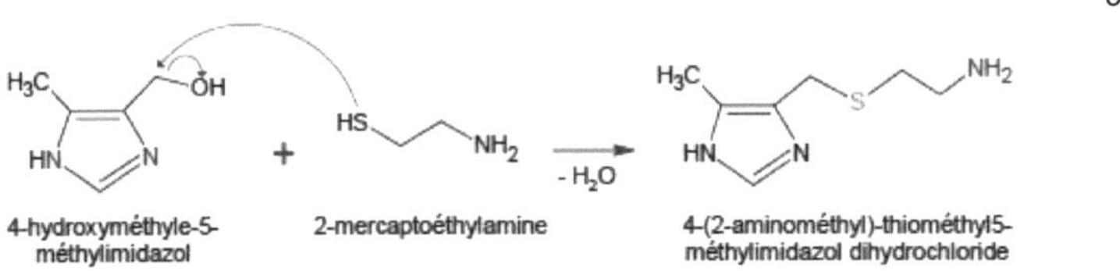

Figure 21. Chemical synthesis of cimetidine (continued).

4- 4-(2-aminomethyl)-thiomethyl5-methylimidazol dihydrochloride reacts with N-cyanimido-S,Sdimethyldithiocarbonate to give a thiourea derivative, which is converted to cimetidine by reaction with methylamine.

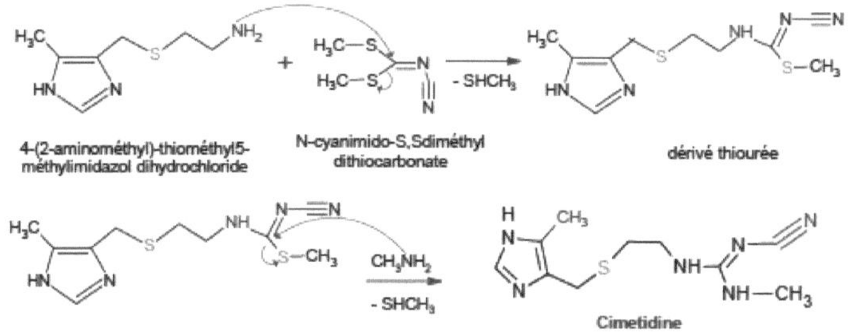

Figure 22. Chemical synthesis of cimetidine (continued).

7.1.2. Analytical control

1. Physico-chemical properties

Cimetidine is a white or approximately white powder. It is sparingly soluble in water, soluble in 96% ethanol and practically insoluble in methylene chloride. Cimetidine dissolves in dilute mineral acids. Cimetidine is polymorphic.

2. Identification

- Melting point: 139°C to 144°C.
- Infrared absorption spectrophotometry
- Thin layer chromatography
- Atropine sulphate gives the alkaloid reaction

3. Test

- Appearance of the solution
- Related substances
- Loss on drying
- Sulphuric ash

4. Dosage

Titration by potentiometry.

7.2. Business structure relationship

In the search for a selective H2 receptor antagonist, the structure of histamine was used as a chemical starting point.

Chemical studies conducted on the latter suggest that tautomerism of the imidazole ring of histamine may be involved as a proton transfer agent, so the first H2 receptor antagonists were imidazole derivatives, and burimamide was the first to be examined in humans.

Chemical modification of this drug led to metiamide (Black et al. 1973) and cimetidine (Brimblecombe et al. 1975).

Initially, it was thought that the imidazole part of the molecule was essential for its histamine H2 receptor antagonist properties, but it later emerged that other 5-membered rings, such as furan and thiazole, also fulfilled these criteria.

Recently, the 5-membered ring has been replaced by a phenyl group in the H2 receptor antagonist roxatidine.

Despite their great diversity, all known H2-receptor antagonists comprise an aromatic ring with **a flexible chain of 4 atoms** linked to **a polar group** (aromatic ring - flexible chain - polar group).

These compounds can be grouped into 4 main series according to the nature of the aromatic rings, namely the imidazole (cimetidine), dimeihylaminofuran (ranitidine), guanidino-thiazole (famotidine) and piperidinomethylphenoxy (roxatidine) series.

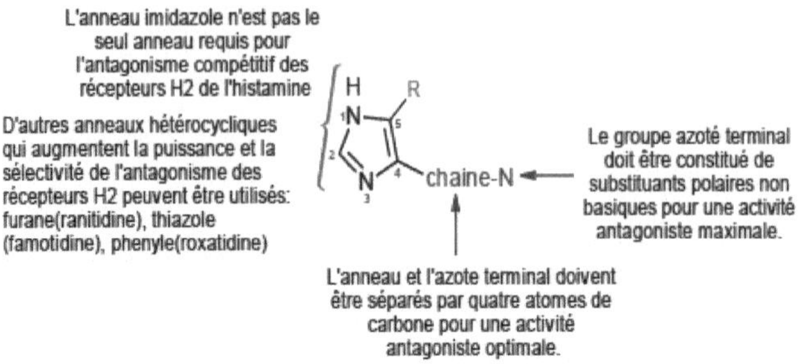

L'anneau imidazole n'est pas le seul anneau requis pour l'antagonisme compétitif des récepteurs H2 de l'histamine

D'autres anneaux hétérocycliques qui augmentent la puissance et la sélectivité de l'antagonisme des récepteurs H2 peuvent être utilisés: furane(ranitidine), thiazole (famotidine), phenyle(roxatidine)

H R
N
N
chaine-N

Le groupe azoté terminal doit être constitué de substituants polaires non basiques pour une activité antagoniste maximale.

L'anneau et l'azote terminal doivent être séparés par quatre atomes de carbone pour une activité antagoniste optimale.

The imidazole ring is not the only ring required for competitive antagonism of histamine H2 receptors
Other heterocyclic rings that increase the potency and selectivity of H2 receptor antagonism can be used: furan (ranitidine), thiazole (famotidine), phenyl (roxatidine), etc.
The terminal nitrogen group must be made up of polar, non-basic substituents for maximum antagonistic activity.
The ring and terminal nitrogen must be separated by four carbon atoms for optimum antagonistic activity.

Figure 23. Structure-activity relationship between H2 antihistamines.

7.3. Pharmacokinetics

Oral absorption of all the H2-receptor antagonists studied clinically is fairly rapid.
Maximum plasma concentrations are generally reached between 1 and 3 hours after administration, but a second peak has been observed with cimetidine, ranitidine and famotidine.
The average oral bioavailability of H2 antagonists is between 50 and 70%.
All H2 antagonists are eliminated fairly rapidly, with a terminal half-life of 1-3 hours and a total body clearance of 24-48 L/h.
Elimination is mainly by renal excretion, with renal clearances ranging from 13.8 to 30 L/h.

7.4. Indications

- Duodenal ulcers
- Gastric ulcers
- Zollinger-Ellison disease
- Uncomplicated gastro-resophageal reflux disease
- H2-receptor antagonists may also be used off-label for the prophylaxis of stress ulcers, resophagitis, gastritis, gastrointestinal haemorrhage or urticaria.
- These drugs are also sometimes included in a multi-drug regimen for the eradication of Helicobacter pylori.

7.5. Undesirable effects

H2-receptor antagonists are generally well tolerated. Mild side effects may include headache, drowsiness, fatigue, abdominal pain, constipation or diarrhoea.
Use in patients with renal insufficiency, hepatic insufficiency or over 50 years of age has been correlated with side effects on the central nervous system such as delirium, confusion, hallucinations or speech disorders.
Cimetidine is generally considered to be the most frequent cause of these symptoms, although similar effects have also been observed with famotidine.
Drug interactions with H2-receptor antagonists may occur. Due to the therapeutic increase in gastric pH, the absorption of drugs whose dissolution requires an acidic environment may be impaired.
Cimetidine is a powerful cytochrome P450 inhibitor and should be avoided with other drugs metabolised by CYP450 enzymes, such as theophylline, selective serotonin reuptake inhibitors or warfarin.

High and prolonged doses of cimetidine have also been associated with gynaecomastia, reduced sperm count, impotence in men and galactorrhoea in women.

7.6. Contraindications

There is currently no absolute contraindication to H2 blockers.

However, they should not be used in patients with a known hypersensitivity to one of the H2 blockers or to other components of the drug.

8. Conclusion and outlook

Anti-gastric acid drugs play a crucial role in the management of gastrointestinal disorders such as gastro-resophageal reflux disease (GERD), gastric and duodenal ulcers and dyspepsia. These drugs effectively control the production and effects of gastric acid. Each class of drugs offers distinct mechanisms of action, adapted to different clinical conditions.

The outlook for drugs to treat gastric acidity is promising, and focuses on several areas of innovation. The development of new agents with more specific mechanisms of action and improved safety profiles is underway, with the aim of offering more effective and better tolerated therapeutic options. Pharmacogenomics will make it possible to tailor treatments to individual genetic variations, optimising efficacy and minimising side effects. Sustained-release formulations and targeted delivery systems will improve the adherence and efficacy of therapies.

9. References

1. Jadcherla SR, Shaker R: Physiology of aerodigestive reflexes in neonates and adults. In Physiology of the Gastrointestinal Tract, edn 5. Edited by Leonard Johnson. Elsevier; 2012.
2. El-Mahdy, M. A., Mansoor, F. A., & Jadcherla, S. R. (2017). *Pharmacological management of gastroesophageal reflux disease in infants: current opinions. Current Opinion in Pharmacology, 37, 112-117.* [Online]. Available from : Pharmacological management of gastroesophageal reflux disease in infants: current opinions - ScienceDirect.
3. Fofaria, R. K., & Morris, D. L. (2015). *Hiatus hernia and gastroesophageal reflux disease. Medicine, 43(4), 192-196.* [Online]. Available at : Hiatus hernia and gastro-oesophageal reflux disease - ScienceDirect.
4. Slaughter JL, Stenger MR, Reagan PB, Jadcherla SR: Neonatal histamine-2 receptor antagonist and proton pump inhibitor treatment at United States children's hospitals. J Pediatr 2016, 174 63-70.e63.

Salisbury BH, Terrell JM. Antacid. In: StatPearls. Treasure Island (FL): StatPearls Publishing; 2024. [Online]. Available from: https://www.ncbi.nlm.nih.gov/books/NBK526049/.

5. Ahmed A, Clarke JO. Proton Pump Inhibitors (PPI) In: StatPearls. Treasure Island (FL): StatPearls Publishing; 2024. [Online]. Available from: https://www.ncbi.nlm.nih.gov/books/NBK557385/ .
6. Haastrup PF, Thompson W, S0ndergaard J, Jarb0l DE. Side Effects of Long-Term Proton Pump Inhibitor Use: A Review. Basic Clin Pharmacol Toxicol. 2018 Aug;123(2):114-121. [Online]. Available from: Side Effects of Long-Term Proton Pump Inhibitor Use: A Review - PubMed (nih.gov).
7. Mears JM, Kaplan B. Proton pump inhibitors: new drugs and indications. Am Fam Physician. 1996 Jan;53(1):285-92. [On-line]. Available from: Proton pump inhibitors: new drugs and indications - PubMed (nih.gov).
8. Shin, J. M., & Sachs, G. (2004). *Proton Pump Inhibitors. Encyclopedia of Gastroenterology, 259-262.* [On-line]. Available from: Proton Pump Inhibitors - ScienceDirect.
9. Shaw, D. H. (2017). *Drugs Acting on the Gastrointestinal Tract. Pharmacology and Therapeutics for Dentistry, 404-416.* [Online]. Available from: Drugs Acting on the Gastrointestinal Tract - ScienceDirect.

10. Wermuth, C. G., Villoutreix, B., Grisoni, S., Olivier, A., & Rocher, J.- P. (2015). *Strategies in the Search for New Lead Compounds or Original Working Hypotheses. The Practice of Medicinal Chemistry, 73-99 [**Online**]. Available on :* Sci-Hub | Strategies in the Search for New Lead Compounds or Original Working Hypotheses. The Practice of Medicinal Chemistry, 73-99. | 10.1016/b978-0-12-417205-0.00004-3

11. Vardanyan, R. S., & Hruby, V. J. (2006). *Antihistamine Drugs. Synthesis of Essential Drugs, 219-235. [**On line**]. Available on :* Sci- Hub | Antihistamine Drugs. Synthesis of Essential Drugs, 219-235 | 10.1016/b978-044452166-8/50016-9

12. European Directorate for the Quality of Medicines and Healthcare. Sodium bicarbonate monograph. **In**: *European Pharmacopoeia*. 9th ed. France: EDQM, 2018, p. 3820.

13. European Directorate for the Quality of Medicines and Healthcare. Omeprazole product monograph. **In**: *European Pharmacopoeia*. 9th ed. France: EDQM, 2018, p. 3433-3434.

14. European Directorate for the Quality of Medicines and Healthcare. Misoprostol product monograph. **In**: *European Pharmacopoeia*. 9th ed. France: EDQM, 2018, p. 3296-3297.

15. European Directorate for the Quality of Medicines and Healthcare. Cimetidine monograph. **In**: *European Pharmacopoeia*. 9th ed. France: EDQM, 2018, p. 2237-2239.

Chapter 4

Laxatives

1. Introduction

The term "laxative" covers all substances that encourage defecation. In reality, it is often reserved for drugs, most of which have a sudden action, resulting in the evacuation of more or less moulded stools.

Laxatives are widely used in the treatment of constipation and the vast majority are available over the counter without a prescription.

2. Pathophysiological background

Constipation is a common functional gastrointestinal disorder. It affects around 20% of the world's population. It is much more common in women and the elderly.

In addition, constipation can have several aetiologies (organic or functional).

2.1. Definition

The World Organisation for Gastroenterology defines constipation as: "A condition characterised by persistent difficulty with defecation or a sensation of incomplete exoneration and/or infrequent defecation (less than 3 times per week), in the absence of alarm symptoms or secondary causes".

Because of these varying definitions, an international panel of gastroenterology experts established certain criteria to define constipation. "The overriding aim was to classify functional gastrointestinal disorders (FGIDs) using a symptom-based classification scheme, emphasising that patients report symptoms". In fact, the patient must experience at least 2 of the following criteria and/or symptoms for at least three months out of if.

- Efforts to defecate in more than 25% of defecations;
- Hard or lumpy stools in more than 25% of bowel movements;
- Feeling of incomplete exoneration in more than 25% of bowel movements;
- Sensation of anorectal blockage in more than 25% of bowel movements;
- Manual manoeuvres facilitate exoneration in more than 25% of bowel movements;
- Less than three bowel movements a week

2.2. Types of constipation

Physiological defecation is a fairly complex process. Constipation disorders can have several origins. Skardoon and colleagues (Skardoon et al., 2017), have thus been able to identify subtypes of constipation:

— Normal transit constipation, also known as "functional constipation"; this is the most common type in the population;

— Slow transit constipation: transit time is prolonged;

— Pelvic floor dyssynergia is a sensation of obstruction when passing stools. This is due to a coordination problem between the abdominal muscles and the pelvic floor muscles.

2.2.1. Occasional constipation

Occasional constipation is a separate entity. The patient complains of constipation which appears quite suddenly in particular circumstances such as the last months of pregnancy, bed rest or travelling.

2.2.2. Secondary constipation

It can have both extra-digestive and digestive causes.

2.2.3. Iatrogenic constipation

Many medicines can cause constipation:

— Opiate addiction, chronic occupational or domestic poisoning by lead or arsenic;

— Long-term treatment with anticholinergics, barbiturates, antidepressants, neuroleptics, hypotensive drugs (especially calcium antagonists), diuretics and iron salts.

2.2.4. Functional constipation

Functional constipation is generally described as a condition characterised by persistent difficulty with defecation or a sensation of incomplete exoneration and/or infrequent defecation (once every three to four days or less) in the absence of alarm symptoms or secondary causes.

Motor disorders

Motor disorders are generally due to a lengthening of the transit time.

Intestinal transit time is generally 36 to 48 hours. However, this time varies depending on the region of the intestine. On average, "the duration of intestinal transit is a few seconds or minutes in the resophagus, 30 minutes to two hours in the stomach and one to four hours in the small intestine, the remaining time being that of colonic transit".

The digestive tract is unique in that it has its own nervous system. In order to have contractile activity, the digestive tract has smooth muscle cells. It also has secretory cells. Within the digestive wall there are two major plexuses that form the enteric nervous system. These are the enteric submucosal plexus, also known as Meissner's plexus, and the myenteric plexus, also known as Auerbach's plexus.

We find other types of cells close to the plexuses: these are Cajal's interstitial cells (CIC). They are found between the layer of longitudinal and circular muscle fibres (within the submucosa). These cells are connected to other smooth cells (Meissner's plexus) by tight junctions forming a nerve network. Alteration of Cajal's interstitial cells will lead to a decrease in CPHA and therefore induce constipation.

3. Laxatives

A laxative is a medicine used eliminate soft but formed faeces.

Depending on the dose administered, the laxative may have a purgative action, i.e. it will cause watery evacuation, or a more irritative action, which may be associated with stomach cramps and/or electrolyte loss.

Treatment for habitual constipation is based on dietary hygiene rules (physical activity, high-fibre diet), possibly combined with a lubricant laxative.

There are five families of laxatives:

— Osmotic laxatives ;

— Ballast laxatives ;

— Lubricating laxatives ;

— Stimulant laxatives ;

— Rectal laxatives.

4. Osmotic laxatives

By generating an osmotic gradient, osmotic laxatives act by retaining water in the colonic lumen, which will lead to an increase in faecal volume and possibly increase digestive contact, although this latter mode of action has never been proven in constipated patients.

There are sweet osmotic laxatives and salty osmotic laxatives.

> Sweet osmotic laxatives

These are sugars that are not absorbed by the intestine. They include lactulose

(*DUPHALAC®*) and lactitol (*PIZENSY®*)(5).

Salty osmotic laxatives

Saline laxatives consist of salts dissolved in a liquid; they quickly eliminate all the contents of the intestines. They usually work between 30 minutes and 3 hours. Examples include salts of citric acid (*ROYVAC®*), magnesium oxide (*CITRAFLEET®*) and magnesium hydroxide *(CHLORUMAGENE®)*.

> Pure osmotics

This is polyethylene glycol (PEG) or macrogol (Forlax®), a non-absorbable substance.

Macrogols increase the number of bowel movements (an increase of 1.98 bowel movements/week compared with placebo, and 1 bowel movement/week compared with lactulose), reduce their consistency and reduce the need to push.

Table I. Main osmotic laxatives.

Molecule DCI	Trade name and form pharmaceutical	Chemical structure and scientific name
Lactulose	***DUPHALAC®*** Suspension buvable sirop	**4-O-β-D-galactopyranosyl-D-fructose**
Lactitol	***PIZENSY®*** Poudre pour solution buvable	**4-O-β-D-Galactopyranosyl-D-glucitol**
L'hydroxyde de magnésium	***CHLORUMAGENE®*** Poudre orale 100g	OH^- Mg^{2+} OH^-
L'oxyde de magnésium	***CITRAFLEET®*** Poudre pour solution buvable 3,5g	O^{2-} Mg^{2+}
Polyéthylène glycol	***Forlax®*** Sachet 10g	

4.1. Study of the lead manager

Lactulose: *DUPHALAC®*

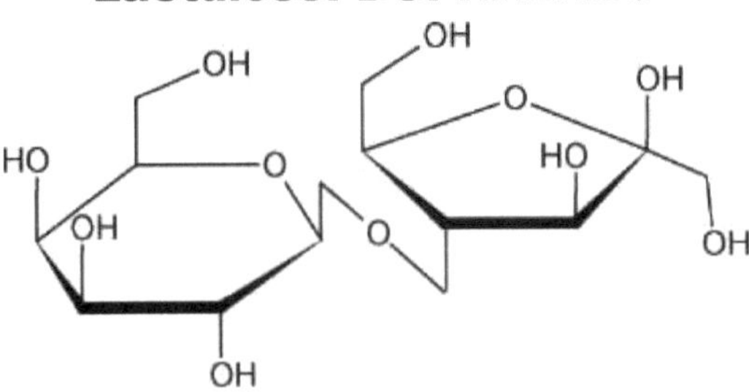

Figure 1: Lactulose structure.

4.1.1. Chemical synthesis

Lactulose is produced industrially exclusively by the chemical isomerisation of lactose via the deLobry de Bruyn-Alberda van Ekenstein (LA) rearrangement, which can be summarised as the formation of an enol intermediate of lactose and epilactose in an alkaline medium, with the transformation of the glucose of the lactose molecule into fructose, resulting in the lactulose molecule.

Conventional preparation of lactulose involves adding an alkaline agent such as $Ca(OH)_2$, KOH, K_2HPO_4 $Ba(OH)_2$, 8 H_2O, etc., to a solution of lactose. The solution is heated and the time required for the two isomers to equilibrate varies from 10 minutes to 2 days depending on the temperature: 30°C to 130°C.

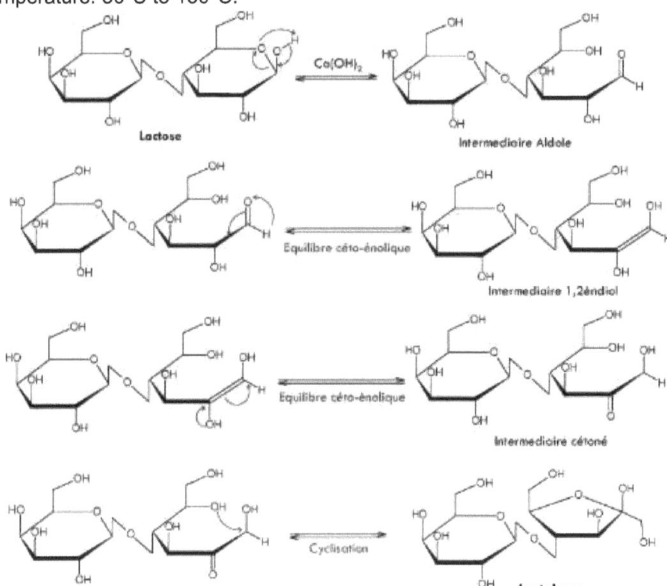

Figure 2. Lactulose synthesis.

4.1.2. Analytical control

1. Physico-chemical properties

Lactulose is a clear, viscous, colourless or pale yellow-brown liquid. It is miscible with water.

2. Identification

- Thin layer chromatography
- To 0.1 g of liquid lactulose, add 10 mL of water R and 3 mL of cupri-tartaric solution R, then heat. A red precipitate forms.
- To 0.25 g of liquid lactulose, add 5 mL of water R and 5 mL of ammonia R. Heat in a water bath at 80°C for 10 min. A red colour develops.

3. Test

- Related substances
- Loss on drying

- Sulphuric ash

4. Dosage

Liquid chromatography

4.3.3. Pharmacokinetics

After oral administration, less than 3% of a given dose of lactulose solution is absorbed by the small intestine.

It is mainly metabolised in the colon by the saccharolytic bacteria present there. In particular, the substance is broken down into lactic acid and small quantities of acetic and formic acid.

Renal excretion of lactulose has been determined to be less than or equal to 3% and is generally complete within 24 hours. Unabsorbed lactulose is largely excreted in the faeces.

4.3.4. Indications

Lactulose is indicated as a laxative in the **treatment of chronic constipation** in adults and geriatric patients. Lactulose is also **used as an adjunct to protein restriction** and supportive therapy for the prevention and treatment of portosystemic encephalopathy (PHE), including variants of hepatic pre-coma and coma.

5. Ballast laxatives

They include dietary fibre, known as insoluble fibre, and mucilage, known as soluble fibre because it is made of a substance that swells on contact with water. They make the stools denser and more voluminous, and cause them to retain more water, which encourages natural peristalsis and therefore their progress. They speed up colonic transit in two to three days.

This is the case with psyllium (*PSYLIA®*, *PSYLLIUM®*), ispaghul tegument (*SPAGLULAX®*, *TRANSILANE®*) and sterculia gum (*NORMACOL®*).

6. Lubricants

Lubricants are absorbed orally. They act by a mechanical effect that (modestly) facilitates the progress of stools through the intestine, by sliding, and water absorption. They take effect in six to eight hours.

They are represented by paraffin oil and are indicated in constipation in failure (primary/secondary) of osmotic/mucilage type laxatives.

Mineral oil, or paraffin oil, is a mixture higher alkanes derived a mineral source, such as petroleum. Petroleum mineral oil is made from crude oil by vacuum distillation to produce several distillates and a residual oil, which are then refined.

7. Stimulant laxatives

Stimulant laxatives work by increasing colonic motricity and therefore promoting the progress of bowel movements.

Stimulant laxatives increase intestinal motricity and secretions.

They should be used for the short-term treatment of occasional constipation to avoid addiction.

> Anthraquinone (anthracene) heterosides :

- Senna powder.
- Cascara extracts.
- Senosides.

> Castor oil

> Phenylmethane derivatives :

- Bisacodyl.
- Sodium picosulphate.

Table II. Main stimulant laxatives.

Molecule INN	Trade name and pharmaceutical form	Chemical structure and scientific name
Bisacodyl	***DULCOLAX®*** Comprimé 5/10 mg	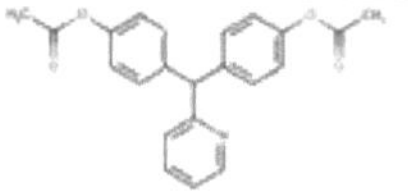 4,4'-(pyridin-2-ylmethyle ne)bis(phenyl)dibutyrate
Picosulfate de sodium	***CLENPIQ®*** Solution buvable 10 mg/160mL	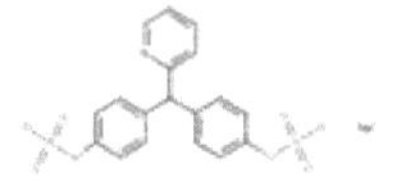 (4-(2-(1,2-dioxo-1,2-dihy dro-3H-indol-3-yl)ethy l)phenyl) hydrogen sulfate

7.1. Study of the lead partner

Bisacodyl: *DULCOLAX® (in French)*

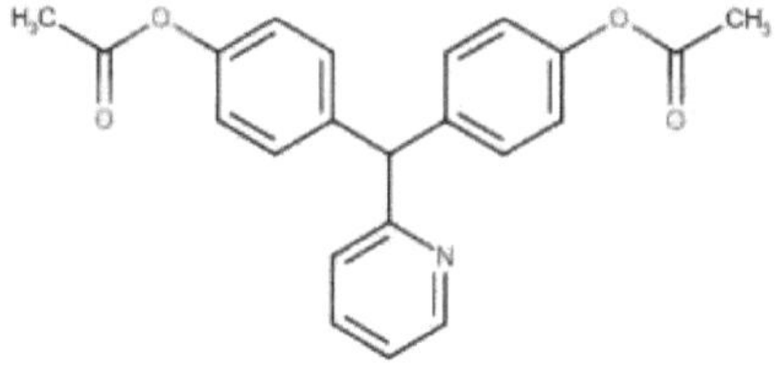

Figure 3: Structure of bisacodyl.

Bisacodyl is a phenolphthalein activated by an enzyme in the ileal and colonic mucosa (endogenous deacetylase).

Bisacodyl, a diphenylmethane derivative, is a stimulant laxative used for the temporary relief of occasional constipation and colon cleansing in preparation for colonoscopy in adults.

Bisacodyl is thought to act directly on the nerve plexus of the colonic mucosa. It takes effect in six to eight hours, and can be administered orally or rectally.

7.1.1. Chemical synthesis

Bisacodyl is synthesised from pyridine-2-carbaldehyde and phenol by an electrophilic addition reaction in acid medium, followed by an acetylation reaction with acetic anhydride.

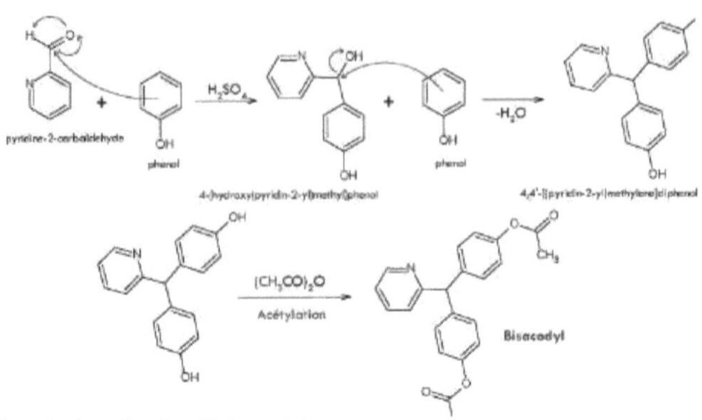

Figure 4: Chemical synthesis of bisacodyl.

7.1.2. Analytical control

1. Physico-chemical properties

Bisacodyl is a white or almost white crystalline powder. It is practically insoluble in water, soluble in acetone and fairly soluble in 96% ethanol.

2. Identification

- Melting point: 131°C to 135°C.
- Ultraviolet and visible absorption spectrophotometry.
- Infrared absorption spectrophotometry.
- Thin layer chromatography

3. Test

- Related substances
- Sulphuric ash
- Acidity or alkalinity
- Loss on drying

4. Dosage

Potentiometric titration with perchloric acid.

7.1.3. Pharmacokinetics

Bisacodyl is deacetylated to active bis-(p-hydroxyphenyl)-pyridyl-2-methane (BHPM) by intestinal deacetylase. A small amount of BHPM is absorbed from the gastrointestinal tract and glucuronidated being eliminated.

The majority of bisacodyl is eliminated in the faeces.

8. Rectal laxatives

Local laxatives are treatments introduced via the anal route. Depending on their presentation, they act at rectal, recto-sigmoidal or even left colonic level.

They take the form of suppositories or enemas. The aim is to make the stool pass after a few minutes (usually 5 to 30 minutes).

8.1. Suppositories

They are used to empty the rectal reservoir, the two main active ingredients most commonly used being :

- Effervescent suppositories potassium tartrate and sodium bicarbonate (such as *EDUCTYL®*). The volume of carbon dioxide released in the rectum increases intra-rectal pressure and triggers the exonerative reflex.

- Glycerine suppository made from glycerol, which stimulates peristaltic movements, reduces water resorption and helps with reflex defecation.

8.2. Washing

They soften the stool and trigger a contraction of the rectum to evacuation. They allow the rectum and part of the sigmoid colon to be emptied. The main enemas used are :

— *MICROLAX LAVEMENT®:* 5 ml single-dose rectal solution for adults and 3 ml for babies, containing sodium citrate, sodium lauryl sulphoacetate and 70% sorbitol.

— *NORMACOL LAVEMENT®:* single-dose rectal solution whose active substance is sodium dihydrogen phosphate dihydrate and sodium hydrogen phosphate dodecahydrate.

8.3. Study of the lead partner

Glycerol: *GLYCERINE®*

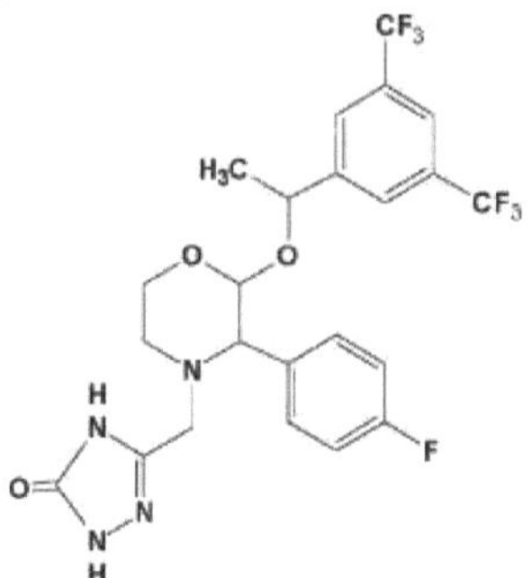

Figure 5. Structure of Glycerol.

8.3.1. Chemical synthesis

Glycerol is synthesised from propene by an allylic (radical) substitution reaction with dichlor at 773K, followed by a nucleophilic substitution reaction with sodium hydroxide to form prop-2-en-1-ol, followed by a nucleophilic addition reaction with hypochlorous acid and finally a nucleophilic substitution reaction with sodium hydroxide to form glycerol.

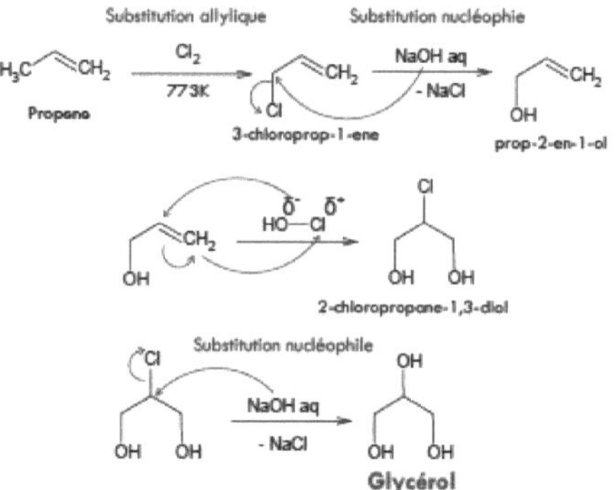

Figure 6. Chemical synthesis of glycerol.

8.3.2. Analytical control

1. Physico-chemical properties

Glycerol is a syrupy liquid, smooth to the touch, colourless or almost colourless, clear and very hygroscopic. It is miscible with water and 96% ethanol, sparingly soluble in acetone and practically insoluble in fatty oils and essential oils.

2. Identification

- Refractive index
- Infrared absorption spectrophotometry

3. Test

- Related substances
- Sulphuric ash
- Water

4. Dosage

Titration by potentiometry.

9. Mechanism of action

9.1. Osmotic laxatives

These substances have a purely physical mode of action: they are not absorbed by the body and are excreted unchanged.

They increase the hydration of the stools through a phenomenon known as "*osmosis*", *in* other words the drawing in of water from the colon, the lower part of the intestine. Stools then become more abundant, softer and easier to evacuate.

Sugar laxatives are absorbed in the colon, resulting in water retention. This water retention increases the hydration of the stools and therefore their volume. It is the metabolisation of the molecules that causes undesirable effects, such as flatulence and abdominal pain.

Saline laxatives attract and retain a large volume of isotonic fluid in the stomach. This stimulates peristalsis in the small intestine, reducing transit time and triggering watery stools.

9.2. Ballast laxatives

They include dietary fibre, known as insoluble fibre, and mucilage, known as soluble fibre because it is made from a substance that swells on contact with water.

The effect of fibre on transit has been known since the time of Hippocrates. This is the case with the bran (the husk) of cereals, found in wheat, oats, rice, etc. Fibre increases faecal volume while softening the stool, making it easier and quicker to expel.

Mucilages have hygroscopic properties and are capable of absorbing and retaining large quantities of water, up to twenty times their weight. They hydrate faeces and increase their volume. The resulting mechanical distension stimulates peristalsis and facilitates the passage of faecal matter.

9.3. Lubricating laxatives

These are mineral oils, derived from petroleum. This is particularly true of paraffin oil, which softens faeces by delaying the absorption of water from the stool and lubricating the digestive tract.

They take effect in six to eight hours. They are used in situations where the patient has difficulty "forcing" or "pushing", such as after heart or digestive surgery or haemorrhoYdectomy.

Taking lubricating laxatives can alter absorption of fat-soluble vitamins A, D, E and K. This is why they should not be taken continuously to avoid vitamin deficiencies. There is also a risk of inhalation pneumonitis if users lie down in the minutes following administration.

9.4. Stimulant laxatives

It can be of plant origin, such as senna (*PURSENNIDE®*), or chemical, such as bisacodyl (*DULCOLAX®*).

Their recommended duration use is short, ten days maximum. intensity of their action varies according to the dose taken, and may lead to significant purging with electrolyte loss. Possible side effects with this class are abdominal pain and cramps, and diarrhoea. In addition, problems of tolerance and habituation may occur long-term use.

9.5. Rectal laxatives

Enemas and suppositories These have a very rapid local action. They are indicated for terminal constipation, in preparation for an X-ray examination or to prevent the patient from "straining" after surgery or childbirth.

Enemas empty the distal colon by distension. Following an enema, the resulting faecal evacuation varies between 0.1 and 2.8 kg, with a median weight of 1.2 kg.

There are also different classes of laxatives in suppository form. Glycerine, for example, is an osmotic laxative which, in suppository form, triggers defecation through its hygroscopic, rectal dilating and irritant action. There are also stimulant laxatives in suppository form, such as Bisacodyl (*DULCOLAX®*).

10. Conclusion and outlook

Laxatives are pharmacotherapeutic agents used to treat constipation by facilitating intestinal movements. They are divided into several main classes, each with a specific mechanism of action. Although these drugs are effective, they must be used with care to avoid side effects such as dependence, electrolyte imbalances and dehydration.

The future of laxative pharmacotherapy could benefit from a number of advances. Firstly, the development of new targeted laxatives, based on a better understanding of the molecular mechanisms of constipation, could reduce side effects and increase efficacy. Research into the intestinal microbiome paves the way for personalised treatments, adapted to patients' specific microbial profiles, to improve the management of constipation. In addition, combined formulations, incorporating prebiotics or probiotics with laxatives, could offer additional benefits by favourably modifying the intestinal microbiota.

11. References

1. JOHNSON, Leonard R. *Physiology of the gastrointestinal tract.* Elsevier, 2006. [On-line]. Available from: Physiology of the Gastrointestinal Tract - Google Books
2. KLASCHIK, E., NAUCK, Friedemann, and OSTGATHE, C. Constipation-modern laxative therapy. *Supportive care in cancer*, 2003, vol. 11, p. 679-685. [On-line]. Available from: Constipation- modern laxative therapy | Supportive Care in Cancer (springer.com).
3. CAMARA, B. M. La constipation. *Médecine d'Afrique Noire*, 1999, vol. 46, no 4, p. 244-247. [On line]. Available from: 44613.pdf (santetropicale.com).
4. BINDER, Henry J. Pharmacology of laxatives. *Annual review of pharmacology and toxicology*, 1977, vol. 17, no. 1, pp. 355-367. [On line]. Available from: Pharmacology of Laxatives | Annual Reviews
5. Talbert M, Willoquet G, Calop J, Gervais R. Le guide pharmaco clinique .Le Moniteur des pharmacies - Wolters Kluwer France; 2009. [On online].Available on: https://books.google.dz/books?id=dBybk
6. SABATÉ, J. M. and JOUÊT, P. Traitements laxatifs. *book produced with the participation and support of*, p. 63 [On line]. Available from:.livre- RCP-consti2017long.pdf (snfcp.org)
7. Johnson CD, Budd J, Laxatives after hemorrhoidectomy. Ward AJ.Dis Colon Rectum.

1987 Oct;30(10):780-1.
8. COFFIN, B. Gentle laxatives. *Colon & Rectum*, 2009, vol. 1, no 3, p. 3537. [On-line]. Available at:..Mild laxatives (infona.pl).
9. European Directorate for the Quality of Medicines and Healthcare. Lactulose monograph. **In**: *European Pharmacopoeia*. 9th ed. France: EDQM, 2018, p. 3073-3075.
8. European Directorate for the Quality of Medicines and Healthcare. Bisacodyl monograph. **In**: *European Pharmacopoeia*. 9th ed. France: EDQM, 2018, p. 1996-1998.
9. European Directorate for the Quality of Medicines and Healthcare. Glycerol monograph. **In**: *European Pharmacopoeia*. 9th ed. France: EDQM, 2018, p. 2820-2821.

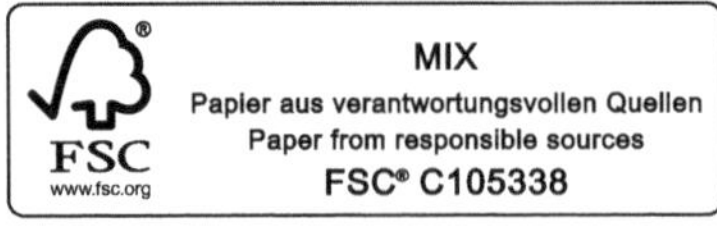

Printed by Books on Demand GmbH, Norderstedt / Germany